DI RECOVERY

2

Restoring Mind and Metabolism from Dieting, Weight Loss, Exercise, and Healthy Food

By Matt Stone

A proud presentation of:

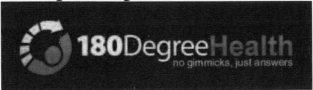

May 2013
Copyright © 2013 180DegreeHealth, LLC. All rights
reserved worldwide.
ISBN 1483922146
ISBN-13: 978-1483922140

DISCLAIMER

The material provided here is for educational and informational purposes only and is not intended as medical advice. The information contained in this book should not be used to diagnose or treat any illness, metabolic disorder, disease, or health problem. If you have developed a serious illness of some kind, the complexities of dealing with that disorder are best handled by your physician or other professional health care provider, whom you should also consult with before beginning any nutrition or exercise program. Use of the programs, advice, and other information contained in this book is at the sole choice and risk of the reader.

When reading this remember that one book cannot be everything for everyone. Only you can decide for yourself what feels right, and ultimately what serves you. Your health is YOUR experiment and no one else's. All I can do is plant seeds, open your mind to new ways of thinking and your eyes to new ways of seeing. I hope those seeds grow and flourish in your life and change it in a way that allows you to spend your time here on earth doing what you really want to do.

-Matt Stone; February 2013

Contents

6

Preface

This is a 3rd revision of the book *Diet Recovery*. Well, actually this should be considered more of a dramatic overhaul. Virtually none of the original content from prior editions was preserved. The overhaul ended up being so dramatic that the title of *Diet Recovery II* seemed appropriate.

Prior editions were really meant for an ongoing and pre-established audience, making references to certain things that an ongoing audience understood. This version is about starting from scratch and keeping it very simple and to the point – weeding out as many unnecessary details as possible.

If you are reading a book entitled *Diet Recovery II*, it shouldn't be unreasonable to expect that you…

- Have done several diets in the past, or are currently entrenched in one diet or diet ideology
- Have noticed some drawbacks of forever being on a diet of some kind – some social, some mental/emotional, some physical
- Are generally sick of spending so much precious time and energy obsessing over the tiny details of your diet – which never really seem to yield any major benefits

- Are at least open to the idea that diets can be harmful, and thus be something that one would need to "recover" from
- Are looking for good health and a pretty good way to eat from day to day without being plagued by perfectionism

I bring these up right away so that we are all on the same page and discussing the same thing here. If you are trying to pass certain particular statements made in this book through some kind of litmus test, cross-examining it through some "study" that you've read or wondering WWDAS (What would Dr. Atkins say?) about certain ideas here, then you are not reading the right book.

The major goals of this book are simple…
1)   Help you to rehabilitate your body from the damage that diets do
2)   Help you to rehabilitate your mind from the damage that diets do
3)   Give you some good feedback mechanisms to focus on (metabolic rate mostly) so that you can let your own body guide your health practices rather than having to defer to a guru or expert, or intellectualize every bite of food you eat
4)   Rehabilitate your relationship with exercise and help you strategize better for the physical changes you would like to get from it
5)   Encourage you to put your efforts in life towards something productive instead of relentlessly fixating your mind on your personal appearance/weight/body composition

Thus, *Diet Recovery II* is pretty much what the subtitle suggests: Restoring Mind and Metabolism from

Dieting, Weight Loss, Exercise, and Healthy Food. Add "Restore Self-Esteem" or something like that and, well, you would be reading a book that is EXACTLY what the title suggests it is. Assuming, like, you know – I can write with such focus and not go off on too lengthy of a tangential diversion into some aspect of nutritional minutiae. Hey, it's tough for me too. My name is Matt, and I'm a recovering Health-a-holic. I used to be like you too, reading blogs all over the internet and every book I could get my hands on in pursuit of the perfect diet.

While I haven't thrown the whole baby out with the bathwater, and yes we will talk about a few fundamental aspects of what I've been led to believe is healthy eating, I've still developed the mantra, *"The perfect diet is very unhealthy."* If you don't already, by the end of the book you will know what I mean by that statement.

Believe me, I will try my best not to talk about lectins, phytates, butyric acid, heart rate variability, growth hormone, casein, hormones in the milk, insulin, dopamine receptors, superfoods, or even… (whispers) gluten. Good grief, could I though. I could spin your brain into a concoction like Chef Jake made at Kamp Kikakee – "Eggs Erroneous."

Oh, and please don't be turned off by my sick sense of humor, or greater focus on odd references to 80's trivia (like the reference to *Ernest Goes to Camp* above) than to "double-blind, placebo-controlled studies." If you want a book that focuses on that kind of thing, you are not ready for this book yet. You've still got a lot of learning left to do before you're ready for the unlearning phase.

No really, I'm serious. Intellectual interference between what your body is telling you that you need and what your brain has "discovered" to be the healthiest thing for you to eat (or drink, or do, or ███████ or lay on top of), is a great liability most of the time. And yes, if you must know, there are plenty uh them "study" things that show such a claim is actually verifiable. These studies are done showing the effects of restricted and restrained eating – the most obvious effects showing up when parents interfere with their child's eating. In short, health information is as detrimental, if not more detrimental, than being totally uninformed about what you should and shouldn't eat.

Be certain though, this book is not about giving up on being healthy. Far from it. In fact, the vast majority of people who read this book and implement the ideas here will notice substantial improvements in their overall health, even eating a crappier diet by puritanical eating standards.

This is actually a health book. Very much so. My healthoholism is still active. I've just found that the gods of health are much kinder than I ever expected. They don't expect you to forego eating yummy things, and sometimes sitting around ███ ████ ██ doing nothing instead of doing Tabata burpee sets with your Gymboss is actually quite alright. Yes, you can eat carbs and fats mixed together, in whatever quantity it takes to satisfy your appetite, without intentionally inflicting harm upon yourself somehow to "burn it off" in a hail of guiltfire. Shocking!

Yes, a health book indeed. But it is the path of least resistance to health. You take the minimum effective dose of health consciousness to get the desired effect. You do the things with the highest health reward with the least effort (like getting plenty of sleep and drinking THE RIGHT amount of fluids).

More importantly, the book is written with words like "realistic" and "sustainable" constantly bouncing around in my skull. Sure, I could dazzle you with some 3-month boot camp, carb-cycling, interval training raw vegan macrobiotic gluten-free Paleo detox cleanse. And yeah, you would lose some weight and make some great before and after pics for me to run in an infomercial.

But I don't want to make millions of dollars! ▓▓▓ I had a good month last month and my girlfriend is already telling me we need to upgrade our phones. What? The one I got you last year has booster engines and attachments to be used as a jet pack. Last week you watched *The Goonies* on the ▓▓▓▓ thing in HD while in orbit – all on one charge. And it's not good enough??!! You need an upgrade??!!

No really I don't want my career to culminate in a slow fade into douche-space after a run of infomercials. Nothing against the Gazelle or the equally-astounding "Nutribull▓▓" currently being paraded.

What was I talking about? Oh right. The book.

Yeah, it's awesome man. Just read the thing.

Introduction

Well, I sort of introduced the thing in the preface. I hate it when that happens. Organization, planning, outlines, other cringe-worthy words… They taught me nothing in writing school.

Hi I'm Matt Stone. If this is the first book of mine you've ever read, I would like to apologize in advance. I know my writing can be annoying at times and is not exactly the same voice and standard that you may have seen in other health books. It's not because I'm a complete fool or moron. What I'm really trying to do is keep you awake and on your toes, and allow you to enjoy the experience of learning something interesting and helpful. It's just how I write. Some people love it so much they speaketh of me like a Messiah. Others hate it so much they can't even read the whole thing, and don't take the information I provide seriously.

Well, you win some you lose some I guess. At the very least, I'm having a good time.

More importantly, I want you to know, if you are new to me, that the amount of thought, study, and experience I have is incredibly broad, deep, and vast. You wouldn't really know that just by reading this book, because I want this to be relatively light reading with very straightforward thoughts on the matter at hand.

But I have studied the subject of human health relentlessly, engulfing several hundred books, thousands of studies, blogs, and websites, communicated directly with thousands of people about health matters (my site has over 40,000 comments and counting and I have consulted with several hundred individuals from dozens of countries), and have essentially given myself one of the most complete and in-depth educations on the subject ever accomplished – and I continue to learn and grow at an accelerated rate with each passing year (creeping up on a full decade of full health immersion).

Any diet you've done, I've probably done it. Any book you've read, I've probably read it. Anything you've read on any health subject I've probably read a half dozen opposing viewpoints on it, spent a hundred hours thinking about it, and discussed it with 20 other people. I could very well have written an article or done an audio or video on it too. After all, I have done well over 1,000 at this point on everything from nosebleeds to intestinal bacteria to restless leg syndrome to early puberty. By my best estimates I have written around 5 million words on the topic since 2006 (the equivalent of around 100 novels).

I don't write this to brag, in fact, I'm a little ashamed of such an excess actually. But hopefully it will at least keep you from writing a review saying "Well it looks like anybody can publish a book these days." Yeah man, it's easy. You just have to commit your entire life to studying something for nearly a decade, communicate with hundreds of the world's leading minds in the field of nutrition and health, and write a 5 million word dissertation. Piece of gluten-free cake. Sure, anybody could do that, but only I have.

Wow, okay I've got some issues. Let it go. Deep breath. Count backwards from 10.

What you may be surprised to NOT see in this book is hundreds of studies referenced. This is actually a weak and cheap tactic used by many in the health field to falsely give their theories credibility. This book is not written on Pubmed crutches. Anybody can snoop around Pubmed or something similar looking to validate a theory. It's time-consuming, and fairly pointless, but it looks impressive to those who are blown away by the number of footnotes in front of them.

Sure, I reference a few, but I don't over rely on it. I speak more in terms of basics, common sense, experience (personal and the reports of others), and what just flat-out works. This book is written from the massive amount of knowledge and experience that I have amassed since taking on the health Goliath, which includes a lot more than just cherry-picking meaningless 2-week studies on rodents.

Also, I should mention the fact that I don't have any horse in the race with various claims or beliefs. I have sworn since I first proclaimed myself to be "an independent health researcher launching an investigation into human health" to never sell anything but my information and my information only. I am not an affiliate for any other books or products (unless it includes my own work), I do absolutely no paid advertising for anyone, I will never sell any supplements or anything other than information. I am more of a journalist than I am a health "guru." Well, more of what a journalist ought to be, not how you're thinking of a journalist (cheap, sell-out, talk about any trash that morons will be interested in, overhype stories to get attention, etc.). I mean journalist in the sense that if you found out Anderson Cooper sold Acai capsules after doing a news story on how great it is, you'd never trust another word out of his mouth.

I don't sell Acai berries. I leave that to Dr. Oz.

But even an honest Joe (Mercola) will forever be tainted once putting up a pill, powder, or health gadget for sale. You just can't reliably investigate truth in health matters when you have a financial bias towards something. When researching health, you'll always see what you wanna see when looking at the many points of view on any topic, nutritional or otherwise. So I try not to want to see anything. I just explore with a curious mind. I hope this builds a level of trust between us much tighter than you have with other people who work in this field.

Diet Recovery… A few more words about the intention and history behind this book before we dig in. The genesis of this book can be traced back to early research I did back in 2007, when I first started my foray into the world of metabolism. Early on I thought there was some perfect diet that, if followed diligently enough, would lead to a health happily-ever-after.

But then I came across the book *Solved: The Riddle of Illness* by Stephen Langer and James Scheer. It seemed like a big Armour thyroid infomercial to me at the time, which made me throw up in my mouth a little bit with each page, but the book was still interesting nonetheless. Their focus was on the thyroid, and restoring a proper body temperature to those suffering from a wide array of ailments both minor and major. The book was documenting their rediscovery of the work of pioneer endocrinologist Broda Barnes who I had seen referenced in other books prior.

Broda Barnes was a practicing endocrinologist in the 50's, 60's, 70's, and early 80's in Colorado. He decided to go against the increasingly trendy reliance on blood tests to determine a person's thyroid function, and decided instead to focus on the outwardly metabolic rate as a whole. He did this very simply, he just had people take their body temperatures first thing in the morning. Those below 97.8 degrees F, who also presented with symptoms congruent with what was known about a low metabolic rate, were treated to get body temperature back up to around 98 degrees F or above (he used armpit/axillary temperature, which runs about a half degree below oral temperatures, and nearly a full degree below ear or rectal temps).

And, eventually, I devoured the entire collection of books that Barnes wrote. To this day, they are some of the more impressive works on the topic of human health. Witty, humorous, sharp, and truly groundbreaking. I then dug further, continuing to connect the metabolic rate dots.

But I had a problem with Barnes's work. And Stephen Langer's. And Mark Starr's, author of *Type 2 Hypothyroidism*, and Datis Kharrazian, and Mary Shomon, and Dr. Wilson who coined the term "Wilson's Temperature Syndrome" to describe the low body temperature phenomenon, and Eugene Hertoghe, and Michael Doyle, and popular thyroid websites such as Stop the Thyroid Madness.

They all looked at a low metabolic rate…
1. As primarily "genetic"
2. As a dysfunction of the thyroid gland, mostly

X 3. As something in need of medication to correct

I was not satisfied with that. The point of my health investigation was not to conclude that everyone needed to be dependent on their doctors and pharmacists to solve their problems. Rather, the whole point and mission of my research is to discover root causes of health problems and practical, do-it-yourself ways to prevent and sometimes even reverse your ailments. So, although I genuinely believe that ALL of the above-mentioned people have helped or are helping a lot of people, and I believe they are generally on track with what is a big medical breakthrough, I couldn't help but ask a bigger fundamental "why" about the peculiar modern phenomenon of having a below-normal body temperature (it's actually been acknowledged that global average body temperature is in decline – even the *New York Times* wrote an article entitled "Rethinking 98.6").

The journey deeper led me to pioneers in the field of nutrition for starters, who had showed that there was something peculiar about the modern diet in terms of its ability to alter our physiology on a really fundamental level. Everyone has their theory as to why, but it doesn't always add up, perhaps because, as humans, we are such complex psychological and emotional beings, and perhaps because we are so phenomenally adaptable.

That's a deep rabbit hole, and we will touch very lightly on that in this book. Suffice it to say that the perfect diet, as alluded to earlier, is a wild goose chase at best, and a way to socially isolate and drive yourself mad with information overload at worst. I find it best, on the purely nutrition front, to make a few small changes rather than aim for some primitive, prehistoric, or perfect diet. It's just not realistic or sustainable for many people, nor is it much fun, nor is it particularly effective at improving most people's health.

What I found to be most compelling was seeing how many forms of restricted eating – for health reasons, weight loss, spiritual or moral beliefs, or otherwise, resulted in a noticeably decreased metabolic rate. A little ironically (little meaning a lot in this context), Dr. Atkins summed it up in what has been by far my most overused quote from the tens of thousands of pages I've read over the last decade on the subject of health. In *Dr. Atkins New Diet Revolution* he states (the phrase "this one" referring to his diet program)…

"Remember that prolonged dieting (this one, low-fat, low-calorie, or a combination) tends to shut down thyroid function. This is usually not a problem with the thyroid gland (therefore blood tests are likely to be normal) but with the liver, which fails to convert T4 into the more active thyroid principle, T3. The diagnosis is made on clinical ground with the presence of fatigue, sluggishness, dry skin, coarse or falling hair, an elevation in cholesterol, or a low body temperature. I ask my patients to take four temperature readings daily before the three meals and near bedtime. If the average of all these temperatures, taken for at least three days, is below 97.8 degrees F (36.5 C), that is usually low enough to point to this form of thyroid problem; lower readings than that are even more convincing."

Interestingly, Atkins shows his awareness of Broda Barnes's research, acknowledges that any diet or combination of diets can lower metabolic rate, and that there isn't really much wrong with the thyroid gland itself. Brilliant. My observations, study, and experience is absolutely, positively, 100% congruent with the above statement. There is a huge epidemic of reduced metabolic rate sweeping the globe. There is a reason or cause for it, it is often caused and certainly exacerbated by pretty much all of the popular diets and health programs out there, and, through some deductive reasoning and exhaustive experimentation and communication I have come up with a very reliable solution for fixing it. And it gets simpler and simpler the more I learn about what is and is not necessary for correcting this common problem.

And so, this book will go into precise detail about how to figure out if your metabolism is low, and how to fix it if it is. When you do achieve a higher metabolic rate, you will feel many interesting and seemingly-unrelated changes because every system of our body is impacted by the metabolic rate – or the rate at which our cells produce energy.

After discussing a few how's and why's of fixing your metabolism, which goes beyond just recovering from diets (although they are a frequent cause for this suppression of metabolic rate), we'll go on to discussing how to move on from diets in general and move on with your life with health practices you can still feel confident in.

That's about it. Keeping it simple here. I get the headaches from all the deep roots I've put into the groundwork that is my current level of understanding, and you just pick the fruit from the tree.

Before we begin I want to direct your attention once more to metabolism with two short sections – one on the importance of metabolism, and another on the best description I've ever come across on what life as a metabolically-healthy person should feel like. With this focus in mind, you'll have trouble ever going on any stupid diet ever again, because you will immediately recognize the signs of the damage being done.

The Importance of Metabolism

Although my health and nutrition research encompasses many ideas, philosophies, pursuits, and biomarkers of health – metabolism has without a doubt become one of the primary focal points of my investigation. That and 80's movies, particularly those starring Val Kilmer and John Cusack.

Metabolism is a word we generically think of when it comes to weight loss. Metabolism, as we know it, means how many calories we burn per day. Metabolism, as I've come to understand it, is much, much more – and even the words "metabolism" or "metabolic rate" as they are commonly used are misnomers.

For example, if you jog for a couple of hours every day, this is said to raise your metabolism because you are burning more calories through exercise. This is false. Jogging typically lowers metabolism, especially when taken to excess – instead it is the Total Energy Expenditure or TEE that is raised by burning more calories through exercise while the basal metabolic rate or BMR typically drops. If you stop jogging, it is easier to gain fat than ever before because your metabolism has been lowered by this form of exercise. This is just one of the many myths surrounding metabolism.

Another fallacy is that thin people have "high metabolisms," which is sometimes the case, and sometimes not the case at all. All different body types can have an underlying low metabolism. You can store excess fat from a low metabolism, or be incapable of building tissue effectively and suffer from muscle underdevelopment and an emaciated or skinny-fat look.

An increasingly popular myth is the idea that it's good to have a low metabolism – and that if we burn energy more slowly we will live longer. Much of this stems from laboratory research showing that severe calorie restriction (like eating half of what you normally eat) prolongs life in several species like fruit flies, rats, monkeys...

But, like most research, this prolongation of life is taken completely out of context and then turned around and applied to adult humans living and interacting in the real world. It ignores aspects of drastic and game-changing significance like...

1.   The only people successful at permanently reducing calorie intake by at least half are those that develop an eating disorder, the deadliest known psychological disease, which affects 11 million Americans, mostly young women. Statistics I've seen suggest a 25-year reduction of life expectancy once you've been diagnosed with an eating disorder (and dieting/intentional calorie restriction at a young age is the top "risk factor" for developing one).

2.   Humans are surrounded by endless abundance and temptation for food, and with real people in the real world, cutting calories by half leads to massive

rebound hyperphagia (pigging out – as is seen in yo-yo dieting and every human calorie-restriction trial ever conducted).

3.   Calorie restriction experiments are done with animals from birth, which allows their bodies to develop to be smaller in size. When comparing members of the same species, the smaller members usually have a much higher life expectancy than larger members (for example, small dogs live much longer than big dogs, despite radically higher mass-specific metabolic rates). This is a hugely significant difference, and the bodies of the creatures can develop at a rate that makes the low calorie intake sufficient – but this calorie intake is insufficient and causes rapid degeneration when the calorie level is cut after adulthood has already been reached. Comparing calorie restriction from birth to calorie restriction begun in adulthood is a completely invalid comparison.

4.   Calorie-restricted laboratory animals display many characteristics of neurosis, anxiety, and social/behavioral disorders. Thinking that cutting calories will lead to a long and prosperous life in a human is a total fantasy that ignores what science has already shown us.

5.   It may not be the reduction in calories that causes a prolongation of life. Some studies on the restriction polyunsaturated fats (which oxidize and cause aging the fastest), or restricting certain amino acids (like tryptophan or methionine), yield the same

life extension without the restriction of total food intake.

6.   A laboratory is a sterile environment, and even if the calorie-restricted animals lived longer and did have a verifiably slower metabolic rate (pound for pound I don't think they do), it's hard to compare this to the real world. The real world is filled with opportunistic organisms and other pathogens, and a high metabolism controls the strength of the immune system completely. A high body temperature – a result of a high metabolism, protects from invasion just like a fever wipes an infection out. More importantly, it is obvious when looking at the real world what happens when food becomes scarce – famines lead to widespread disease and infection at astronomically higher rates.

The last example we'll use as a springboard into talking about the critical importance of maintaining the highest metabolic rate that you are capable of maintaining for health, infectious and degenerative disease resistance, fertility and sex drive, muscle mass and energy and vigor, high-quality functionality and longevity, and much more.

For starters, we all want to avoid getting sick. Viruses, yeasts, fungi, parasites, and bacteria surround us, and it doesn't take much of a crack in the armor for us to succumb to everything from a common cold or sinus infection to something far more serious. The metabolism is more or less the ultimate protection, and having adequate food supplies in nature protects against widespread epidemics of disease in every species, not just humans. However, when a species outgrows its food supply and no longer has enough food to maintain optimal metabolism, the pathogens quickly take over and disease spreads quickly.

This can all be attributed to a drop in body temperature, which systematically slows down many enzymatic reactions vital to maximal immune system potency as well as many other involved factors. In fact, even a simple drop in body fat levels due to inadequate calorie intake lowers the hormone leptin – the master hormone well-understood to regulate appetite, metabolism, and immune system potency. It also raises the stress hormone cortisol, the primary aging and immunosuppressive hormone.

Of course, you're now thinking "Outgrow our food supply? Humans clearly haven't done that!" And you're right. Food is more abundant than ever, and your typical person is looking to lose fat not gain it. We'll get to that in a minute, but let's say for now that you can have a low metabolism because of a shortage of anything, from lack of sleep to lack of certain nutrients – not just overall calories. And on any given day in the United States for example, 45% of the population reports actively being on some kind of diet – which often triggers the same famine physiology as a real famine.

It's certainly worth pointing out that infectious disease is not just infectious disease. It doesn't just end when the fever and sniffles go away. In fact, I'm a part of a discussion group hosted by researcher and co-author of *The Potbelly Syndrome* (a book showing the countless connections between degenerative disease and infectious agents), Russ Farris, and weekly we receive up to a dozen new studies, articles, and press releases showing new connections between various pathogens and seemingly unrelated diseases. The connections between various pathogens and an endless array of autoimmune diseases, cancers, chronic fatigue, autism, and even heart disease and diabetes are becoming increasingly well-understood. Keeping the immune system optimized by maintaining a high metabolism has ramifications far beyond how many times you have to call in sick at work.

In short, my research has led me down one consistent path. Cellular energy production – what one could call "the metabolism" or "metabolic rate" is central or highly-connected to every known health problem. While raising the metabolism isn't a cure-all for everything, there is no doubt in my mind that with any health problem, the first line of action in overcoming it is getting the metabolism up closer to its ideal range. More importantly, optimizing and guarding the metabolism is the key to preventing illness of all kinds and living life with the maximum number of optimally-functional and disease-free years.

My general rule is that if you have a health problem and a low metabolism, bring the metabolism up first to see if it improves or eliminates the condition. Regardless of the health problem, I believe there is an urgent need to maximize metabolic output for health and well-being in general, so this needs to be addressed no matter what your health problem may be. If that works, great. If it doesn't, THEN you seek out alternative treatments, supplements, medication, and other things to control the issue. The worst case scenario is that you end up with a healthier metabolism, notice at least a handful of health improvements, but still have a lingering problem.

In the rest of this metabolism introduction I hope to lay out just a small sampling of health problems and issues that are directly related to our ability to produce energy.

Constipation

This is a very common disorder. Most people who go daily believe they are not constipated, but really if you are straining at all, spending more than 60 seconds on the toilet, shooting pellets that look like deer poop – you are constipated to some degree. Like most things, it's not black and white where one thing is constipation and everything else isn't constipation. It's more like a scale of 1-10. Bowel movements should occur 1-3 times daily, be moist and full – breaking apart when flushed, easy to expel, low in odor, require little wiping, and so forth.

Metabolism is a primary controller of your bowel transit time, which means the amount of time it takes for the food you ate to come out the other end. A healthy transit time is about 24 hours. The mammal with the lowest metabolic rate is the tree sloth, with a body temperature of 93 degrees F and a transit time of 30 days!!! Lifelong constipation commonly disappears in as little as a couple weeks when metabolism is brought to the ideal level.

Other portions of the digestive system are impacted, pun extremely intended, by the metabolic rate as well. With a high metabolic rate the stomach empties faster causing less gas, bloating, and indigestion, reflux is often eliminated by intensified gastric secretions that occur with a higher metabolic rate (more of the hormone gastrin is released), bacterial overgrowth of the small intestine that occurs in a slow-moving bowel also improves, and the overgrowth is thought to be the predominant cause of IBS – the most common digestive ailment. You get the picture. This is just a small and superficial sampling of how the digestive system is affected by metabolic rate.

Low Energy/Chronic Fatigue

The sloth is a wonderful segue for this topic, as this 93-degree body temperature-havin' hypometabolic creature has extremely low energy levels, low muscle mass, sleeps most of the day, and is well, a sloth! Raising your metabolic rate makes you increasingly less sloth-like. Your energy levels rise, your desire for physical activity rises, the quantity of sleep you need to feel rested decreases (although sleep often improves and deepens to a more youthful, childlike state), drowsiness after meals disappears, and an increase in overall vigor and vitality is the norm.

Low Sex Drive

The metabolic rate controls the rate at which sex hormones like progesterone and testosterone are produced by the body. The higher the metabolic rate, the greater the sex hormone production. The primary hormone responsible for sex drive in men is testosterone, and in women is progesterone. Thus, higher metabolic rate yields increases in testosterone where it was previously lacking, and higher metabolic rate yields greater production of progesterone in women – the hormone of female fertility (progesterone = pro-gestation-hormone). The net result is greater sex drive and sexual performance, as well as ease of building muscle, greater leanness, enhanced athletic ability, and so on.

Amenorrhea/Infertility

Lack of menstrual period, menstrual irregularity and PMS, and female infertility are all generally caused by a lack of progesterone. During the first half of a woman's menstrual cycle (start of period to roughly day 14), estrogen dominates progesterone – meaning there is a much higher ratio of estrogen to progesterone in the body. This stifles the metabolism, which is why women's body temperatures are significantly lower during the first half of the cycle than the second half of the cycle – sometimes by more than .5 degrees F. However, the rise of progesterone stimulates ovulation, a large rise in sex drive typically as well as an increase in vaginal lubrication and other pro-sex changes, and a substantial rise in metabolism.

The metabolism controls the rate at which LDL "bad cholesterol" is synthesized into progesterone. When this happens, lack of menstrual period clears up, and does so very consistently. With this comes improvements in fertility as well as improvements in menstrual symptoms, which usually occur at the end of the cycle if insufficient progesterone is being produced.

High Cholesterol/High triglycerides

As I just mentioned, the metabolism controls the rate at which LDL "bad cholesterol" is converted to progesterone. This is true for a lengthy series of hormones (testosterone in men), not just progesterone. Cholesterol in and of itself is a vital substance, that, if merely swept away with a cholesterol-lowering drug can result in many symptoms – most of which can be attributed to insufficient production of these vital hormones. The answer to high cholesterol is increasing the metabolic rate and turning "bad cholesterol" into vital life-giving, rejuvenating, essential hormones associated with youth and strong disease resistance (I received an email just prior to writing this of a young man who dropped his cholesterol from 220 to 156 following my general guidelines with a rise in "good cholesterol," and he more than doubled testosterone levels). The metabolic rate also controls the rate in which we burn or "oxidize" fats. When metabolic rate is high, triglycerides – blood fats, do not accumulate in the blood. High levels of triglycerides are a prominent risk factor for heart disease.

Heart Disease

Other than the obvious factors listed above, the most successful doctor in the history of medicine at preventing heart disease was Broda Barnes. Barnes took exhaustive and detailed records of his patients, cataloged them, and reported them in official medical studies that he later documented. His patients experienced more than 90% fewer heart attacks than the general public at his time of practice. Only four of over

2,000 patients that he recorded had a heart attack, and each of these four had something out of the ordinary about them – one patient had only been seeing him for a few months, another had just moved away and had discontinued his treatment. He had this great success by making the metabolic rate the sole focus of his practice, having patients keep track of their body temperatures to make sure they maintained a youthful metabolic rate – thus avoiding an elderly disease. He also treated countless health problems using the same protocol. His book, *Solved: The Riddle of Heart Attacks*, which was overlooked by a medical community already entrenched in an ineffective war on cholesterol, has never been challenged on the scientific level – nor have his results as a physician ever been matched.

Cancer

Cancer is a disease of impaired cellular respiration. Many have theorized that the one consistent commonality between all forms of cancer is a lack of sufficient oxygen. When oxygen levels are too low, cells cannot burn glucose for fuel normally, and cancer cells form, which operate under a more primitive type of cell metabolism (anaerobic glycolysis) – converting glucose to lactic acid in the body. Estrogen is the primary anti-respiratory hormone (particularly the type of estrogen called estrone which is produced in the adrenal glands by both men and women), occurring in significant quantities in both genders, that chokes off the oxygen supply to cells. Estrogen is opposed by the hormones of youth such as progesterone and testosterone. Of course, the metabolic rate controls how much of the youth hormones are produced to oppose the anti-respiratory estrogen. As metabolism falls in old age, cancer becomes much more likely. Our best defense is keeping metabolic rate as high as possible, which increases cellular activity, respiration, and cellular oxygenation. There is no better defense against cancer than optimizing and guarding a high metabolic rate.

Conclusion

This was just a small sampling of many of the health problems that have close links to the metabolic rate. Others include all forms of autoimmune disease (the metabolism exerts many direct actions over the thymus gland – our immune system central command), which I've seen dramatically disappear with a rise in metabolism, allergies and asthma which I've seen disappear with a rise in metabolism, sleep disorders, mood disorders, chronic pain, elevated blood sugars or type 2 diabetes, obesity, acne, and countless other issues both minor and major.

While we cannot avoid at least some drop in metabolism as we age, at the very least we can minimize the rate at which it declines. Unfortunately, many accelerate this process with various restricted diets, weight loss attempts, excessive endurance exercise, and many other flawed approaches that slow down the resting metabolism.

The answer is much simpler and easier, and is what most people's bodies are crying for them to do anyhow. And that is get sufficient rest, sleep, and relaxation for starters and pair that with a superabundance of nutritious foods with an emphasis on eating plentiful amounts of what I call the anti-stress S's - starch, sugar, salt, and saturated fat — and more importantly calories. Top this off by spending sufficient time doing enjoyable activities with a little supplemental, well-designed exercise.

I promise you that it is literally impossible to live at your highest level of energy, vitality, resilience, happiness, and health unless you have obtained a reasonably high metabolic rate. And the simplest marker for how well your cells produce energy, and the strength of your metabolism adjusted for size, age, gender, and weight — is none other than the body temperature. Yep, you can test it at home with a $3 thermometer. No crazy blood or hormone panels or other diagnostic procedures or visits to a specialist. Morning temperature ranging from 98.0 to 99.0 degrees F (depending on whether you are testing armpit, ear, forehead, oral, or rectal temperature) is the ideal. Other prominent signs of a healthy metabolism are easily noticeable and detectable with no equipment or numbers at all.

I have taken over 1,000 people to that high metabolic state from dozens of countries — with inferior and outdated versions of this book! So there's hope for you yet Madame Ice Toes and Sir Pees A Lot.

Now let's talk about what a high metabolism feels like…

Markers of an Optimal Metabolic Rate

Yes I have used this lengthy passage excessively in the past. If you have been reading my work for years you're rolling your eyes right now and telling me and Hank to get a room. While body temperature and the warmth of the hands and feet and a handful of indicators are some of the most reliable metrics of how a person's metabolism is functioning, ultimately a well-functioning metabolism reveals itself in just about every physical and even psychological and emotional system one can analyze. Without further ado, here is Henry Bieler's wonderful description of what a healthy person functions like – and ultimately what all diet and lifestyle interventions should aim to inch someone closer toward…

"The physical energy of the adrenal type is seemingly inexhaustible, as is the nervous response of the sympathetic system, a result of perfect oxidation of phosphorous in the nerve tissue. Oxidation of carbon in the muscular system gives the adrenal type his great warmth. Thus, the temperature of his body is scarcely ever below 98.8, with hands and feet always pleasantly warm. As digestion and detoxication of food poisons depend greatly upon oxidation in the liver and intestines, it follows that the typical adrenal type, with his perfect oxidation, has thorough digestion. In fact, he may and often does boast that he can eat any and all

kinds of food without discomfort. The exogenous uric acid products as well as the indoxyl compounds are completely detoxicated in the liver, do not accumulate in the blood, nor are they found in the urine."

"The skeletal muscles are well developed and have splendid tone. Fatigue is practically unknown to the adrenal type. His muscular endurance is spectacular. And the perfect tone of the involuntary muscles is evidenced by complete and rapid peristalsis, resulting in several bowel evacuations daily. He can dine on the most impossible food combinations imaginable with no evil results..."

"The quality of the blood is characteristic. A slight to marked polycythemia (more red cells than usual) occurs; leucopenia, or abnormal white cell count on the low side, is never noted. The blood, which is of a rich, red color, clots quickly. Fatal hemorrhage seldom occurs. The immunity against bacterial invasion is spectacular. The typical adrenal type hardly ever becomes infected, even with venereal diseases..."

"A member of the adrenal-type group has a phlegmatic disposition – easygoing, jolly, slow to anger, never bothered with insomnia, fear or "cold feet." He will often go out of his way to avoid a quarrel. Customarily, he has a wide circle of friends because he is warm-hearted and surrounded by an 'aura' of kindly sympathy."

"Splendid circulation gives him warm, magnetic hands..."

"He never worries...His digestion is good and he is seldom constipated. It is possible for him to stand more treatments, operations and even more lung hemorrhages than any other type of patient. He is the patient most often discharged as arrested or cured. All the treatment necessary for his recovery is supplied by bed rest and fresh air."

To this long list of very accurate characteristics, you could add...

- Healthy sex drive, sexual functionality, and high fertility – both in men and women
- Soft, moist skin – including the hands and lower legs which become dry most easily
- Rapid wound healing
- Infrequent need to urinate, with a rich yellow color even after consuming large amounts of liquid
- Strong, white teeth resistant to decay or sensitivity even consuming large amounts of sweets and rarely brushing
- Regular menstrual cycle with no discomforts, cramps or other symptoms, or PMS
- Fast growing hair and fingernails
- Steady blood sugar, with minimal spikes after meals even with the consumption of rapidly-absorbed carbohydrates
- Ability to go long periods without food without any noticeable discomforts, mood changes, energy changes, etc.
- Moist mouth with abundant saliva even after hours without fluids, and nice pink hue to the tongue

There are many more, some that I'm aware of and many that I have yet to discover. But that is a good overview of what life with an ideal metabolism should feel like. In my experience, these are great indicators to be aware of when assessing the effectiveness of your own dietary and lifestyle practices. Most diets or exercise programs of course require that you adhere to a set prescription no matter what biofeedback you encounter with the idea that it will work out favorably in the end if you follow the guidelines diligently enough.

That's precisely what makes dieting very dangerous and detrimental to a large percentage of people's health who do go the diet route.

Anyway, re-read this section ten times if you need to. Or revisit it from time to time once you've catapulted yourself into the world of genuine health enhancement.

See, this really is a health book, not just a prescription to eat nothing but McNuggets and Sour Patch Kids in a defiant ▓▓▓▓▓▓▓ to the whole concept of diets. There is a middle ground. There is a way to do this intelligently, and to benefit on all fronts – metabolically, psychologically, socially, professionally, and beyond.

But already you should be starting to become aware that there is a lot more to health than just eating the perfect diet, exercising regularly, or being lean. In fact, if you look back throughout many of your dieting escapades you will see that when only focusing on short-term changes in body fat levels or other singular indicators of health, you may have been worsening your functionality in 30 other physical and mental categories. I hope this section helps you bring awareness to more than just your waist circumference or body fat levels (or even cholesterol numbers, blood sugar, blood pressure, etc.) in determining whether or not your health is improving or worsening.

The Problem with the Diet Industry

Most people go on some kind of diet for one of two reasons...

1. To overcome a health problem
2. To lose body fat

That's great and all, but the problem is that the people and organizations in the dieting industry, as well as the medical and alternative health professions...

1. Want to save people from problems they are having
2. Want to be in possession of inside information – be smarter than everyone else
3. Want to make a lot of money
4. Want to change the world and be a hero

People think the dieting industry, or other commercial entities or individuals are all evil and crooked. I really do believe that most of what drives people, not just in the health and dieting industry, but in other fields, are very real and honorable desires that we can all relate to.

Actually, on second thought, those aren't really the problems with the health and dieting industries. The problem is mixing those powerful human drives with not knowing jack ▆▆.

Yes, the problem is that every health and diet professional wants to possess the answers and save people while achieving wealth and heroism, but clear, definitive answers just aren't out there. What people think they know or learn about health is usually just speculation that is downloaded into a diet guru's head and repeated as if it were the gospel descended from the big G.O.D. himself. And it doesn't take much for an individual to convince himself or herself that he or she is changing the world in a positive way.

Here's a saying that I repeat when I have an opportunity to speak in front of large audiences...

"Man I used to know everything about health and nutrition. But then I learned so much I hardly know anything anymore."

Another thing I often say is *"If you aren't confused about health and nutrition then you haven't studied it long enough, or deeply enough."*
That's sort of what I'm getting at here. Everyone wants to have all the answers, and many think that they possess them. The problem is that, as humans, we often believe we have the answer when we don't. Many health gurus are also very resistant and downright vicious towards others that distribute information or advice that is contradictory to their own. I too have been guilty of all of the above many times, but have fortunately outgrown this for the most part.
Yes, when I first started researching and writing about health I was absolutely sure that I knew the answers and really rushed to tell everybody exactly what they needed to do. It wasn't done out of a desire to take advantage of the very vulnerable people out there looking to fix a debilitating health condition or overcome some fat-related personal image crisis. It

wasn't to make bajillions of bucks either, which has never been a very strong motivator. Not at all. I really wanted to help people, and any positive feedback I got convinced me that I was living up to my personal quest to save the world in my own little way.

All this leads to a lot of vulnerable people getting a lot of empty promises and jumping on over-hyped diets, supplements, drugs, and other health protocols with totally naïve expectations.

Hope devouring hype.
And the result is disappointment after disappointment after disappointment, because all health systems and ideologies are wrong in many if not most ways – regardless of how positively sure the health advisor giving out information and products may be, and regardless of how many studies or personal testimonies there are to back up its effectiveness.

You can keep naively believing in the Eternal Life Easter Bunny if you want, but I'm pretty ████ sure the miracle cure you are seeking is not something you're likely to find. If you are on a quest to "find health or die trying," you're more likely to die trying.

I don't want you to give up looking for answers entirely or asphyxiate with cynicism. What's more important is that these ludicrous and increasingly-extreme healthscapades that you may be undertaking are not just empty, but very harmful. And I would wager that they are actually worsening, if not outright causing, many of the health problems that you are experiencing.

So that's the problem with the diet and health industries. They are big on promises and backed by research. Spend enough time immersed in any ideology and it will start to make a ████ lot of sense. They are all very seductive to those with real problems and an irrational desire to solve those problems. But they just don't work, and when you fail your failure is chalked up to some obscure malfunction on behalf of some organ you've never heard of, is "just detox" and part of the process of healing or some other nonsense, or a failure to properly adhere to the recommendations. The worst of course is when your failure results in advice to go to even greater extremes.

"Oh, you were only eating 99% raw. Well then, you are really sensitive to cooked foods. Your diet must absolutely be 100% raw now. No exception!"

"Insomnia and erectile dysfunction on the Paleo diet? What? You ate at a restaurant that serves pasta? You can't just avoid gluten and expect to have perfect health. Even if a plate has served pasta and has gone through the dishwasher 24 times you can still get contaminated! Gluten contamination will get ya. It can take months to clear that tiny bit of exposure out of your system. You must be more strict."

"30 grams of carbs a day and you still have PCOS? You must be really REALLY insulin resistant from all the orange juice you drank as a kid. Well, you know you don't have to eat any carbs at all. The Eskimos only ate fish and meat with no carbs whatsoever and were perfectly healthy up to age 150. In their language there isn't even a word for 'doctor' because they never needed one."

"Not losing weight on 1000 calories per day with an hour of cardio 5 times a week. I see. Have you tried the HCG diet?"

And on and on we could go.

I can assure you that your multiple failures on multiple amazing cure-all programs guaranteed to deliver immortality are not your fault. Your failure is not a fluke. And your health guru isn't even trying to deceive you. He just really wants to believe that Santa Claus does exist, and that he is him! His entire self-worth as a human being is dependent upon his information and theories being right and helping everyone.

When you are ready to get past all these seductive healthy diets, and the seductive logic behind all of them…

"Raw foods are natural. That's what humans were meant to eat and why we are the only sick species."

"Sugar is SOOO bad for you. Sugar consumption has increased by 100 pounds per person per year in the last 200 years! If they put glucose on cancer cells they multiply! It's a toxin!"

"Carbohydrates raise insulin and insulin stores fat. Carbs are the CAUSE of obesity and diabetes. Cut them out of your diet and you will lose weight. It's impossible not to because you are lowering insulin, which makes it impossible for you to store fat."

"Ancestral records show good health of prehistoric man. He didn't have dairy products or grains or fast food, therefore all of the health problems in the world today are from these foods that we simply aren't designed to eat. Remove them and you will heal all disease."

"Our modern animal products are toxic due to poor feeding practices and contaminants in the environment. These new pollutants in our environment are what is causing the big rise in modern diseases. Go vegan and see for yourself as all your health problems go away and you lose weight no matter how much you eat."

…then read on. I won't spend time deconstructing all the diets out there, you'll just have to take it on faith that I know of all of them, have spent real quality time exploring each of them, and have deconstructed the logic and found hundreds of followers telling me the same failure stories.

It's the same thing every time. Either someone fails right off the bat almost from day 1, or they experience a temporary (usually about 6 months) honeymoon period where they are running off of adrenaline with the new diet and feeling like they are on top of the world – meanwhile telling all their friends and family that they have found the Holy Grail of Health (just like the guru does, only he or she set up a business and became financially dependent on the program's success and can't jump ship as easily as you can).

I have dubbed this the "catecholamine honeymoon" (catecholamines are internal stimulant substances that provide a narcotic-level high) that takes place with virtually all of the popular diet and weight loss fads in vogue today…

- Intermittent fasting
- Cleansing and juicing
- Veganism
- Raw foodism
- Low-carb
- Low-calorie
- High volume exercise
- Stimulant drugs/weight loss pills

But this catecholamine rush wears off and what remains is a lot of damage – including the reversal of many health improvements seen during the honeymoon period, and including weight regain if weight is lost. And no, that's not just because people fell off the wagon and binged on pizza and doughnuts (although many hopefully did). I'm talking about weight regain on the exact same diet they lost weight on.

Outspoken critic of restricted eating/dieting Linda Bacon summarized it well in *Health at Every Size*, one of many must-read books for any recovering dieter…

"Commentators often attribute weight regain to people's inability to maintain their diets over the long run: the old 'no willpower' problem. Yet this study was well controlled to support the women in maintaining their diets. Weight regain occurred despite maintaining their reduced-calorie diet! And lest you think these results are particular to low-fat dieting, check out the data from this study to other popular diets. After twelve months, Atkins dieters were eating 289 fewer calories compared to when they started the diet, Zone dieters were eating 381 fewer calories, LEARN dieters were eating 271 fewer calories, and Ornish dieters were eating 345 fewer calories. Yet all were steadily regaining weight over the last six months of the first year. And this despite an accompanying increase in exercise!"

Okay I'm getting bored with this now. I really don't want to exhaustively convince you of something that you are already likely know if you have purchased a book called *Diet Recovery II* – that diets suck, the diet and health industries are 19 parts hype for every 1 part help, and that repeatedly going on diets doesn't work for health enhancement or lasting weight loss (it makes you significantly sicker and fatter, not to mention weirder, don't it?). I want to spend the rest of the book talking in specificity about how you can graduate from highly restrictive eating, stop outsourcing to other people for advice on what to eat, and hopefully help you get your life and health back on track. A big promise full of lots of hype, but I'm gonna try.

Pay attention, because I am right about everything and the following information could really save YOUR LIFE! And all of humanity. And end all crime. And save the polar bears. And impregnate Joan Rivers.

What is Healthy Eating?

A bigger question to ask is what are healthy practices? That question has a relatively simple answer, it's just not something that can be laid out in a fancy bulleted list as part of some breakthrough program. It's something that you can determine on your own, and the way you can do it, as we will discuss at length later on, is to think about it less and pay a lot more attention to your body's biofeedback and internal cues.

Healthy eating is an almost spontaneous result of achieving neutrality with all foods, putting them all on an even playing field. That's a tough thing to do, as most of us, due to the barrage of one-sided information we've exposed ourselves to, leaves us feeling like there are truly healthy foods while others are venomous and downright toxic.

Perhaps some foods really are better than others. But we are not mice in a laboratory. We are complex human beings, and we are also really prone to being dead wrong with our seemingly-genius-at-the-time beliefs about what is and is not good for us. Put another way, we can't just eat the foods from the good list and avoid the foods on the bad list. Ultimately there will be social situations where we will need to be casual about our eating, just relaxing and not worrying about all the ingredients in a dish we are served. Making foods forbidden in our minds also has a way of increasing a primal drive to be naughty and break the very rules we set up for ourselves. I tried for years to eat a perfect diet, but kept bingeing on Krispy Kreme doughnuts – in part because something deep inside felt imprisoned by the dietary laws I had imposed on myself. The other part was that I was freaking starving myself unintentionally and my hunger would escalate the more perfectly I ate until the urge to ingest calorie-dense foods overcame my willpower.

While we are unlikely to ever totally decondition ourselves to what is and isn't healthy, at the very least, I highly recommend the following two tactics…

1. Do not fully restrict anything unless it causes you severe distress soon after ingesting it – even after you have thoroughly attempted to condition and acclimate your body to eating that food

2. Think of health as being something that extends WAY beyond your diet

What I mean in the first tactic, is to not fully abstain from anything unless you feel like you have a truly medical reason for doing so. I don't eat pork for example. It gives me immediate problems, manifesting in chest pain that lasts for several days – even marshmallows or gummi bears will do this to me. Others might have an acute allergic reaction that they haven't found a way to overcome. I definitely don't mean for you to stop strictly avoiding shrimp if they put you into anaphylactic shock. By all means, strictly avoid shrimp!

Rather, if you have been brainwashed to believe something like red meat is unhealthy (a food that is commonly made the villain by health authorities), don't proclaim that you don't eat red meat and that you are a vegan. Just eat less of it instead of avoiding it like a neurotic tightwad. Or let's say you heard that grassfed meat is much healthier than commercial beef. Buy some and eat it at home. Knock yourself out. But don't strictly avoid eating a cheeseburger at a restaurant because the meat is not grassfed. In other words, don't be a perfectionist – one of the traits that readers of this book probably all have in common – certainly the readers of this book that have gotten themselves into really bad shape with strict health practices.

I think as you start to eat more intuitively (eat what you are in the mood for at any given time) and assess your biofeedback and cravings without preconceived notions about a food's relative health merits or faults, you'll get past this tendency. But this is a good way to start to re-enter the world of relatively normal and more importantly – relaxed eating habits.

Speaking of casual and relaxed eating habits, that's part of what I mean by the second tactic – think beyond your diet. Health encompasses many things beyond just what we ingest. Even the act of flip-flopping the consumption of questionably healthy food from an anxiety-inducing event filled with fear into one of sensory enjoyment is enough to completely reverse the health outcome of that meal. Most of my research has led me in the direction of stress as the unified root cause of most illness (stress having a very broad definition that extends way beyond just the psychological aspect of stress). And as I often say, guilt and worry about what you're eating is far more unhealthy than any doughnut I've ever eaten.

Health is a net result of ALL of our thoughts, emotions, social interactions, sleep quantity and quality, hydration levels, and a lot more than just whether the cow you're eating ate grass or corn. In the grand scheme of things, all that dietary small stuff that the healthosphere seems obsessed with is minutiae. Absolute minutiae. Eating grassfed beef to be healthy is like fighting a forest fire with an eye dropper if you aren't sleeping well, hate your life, spend most of your time doing mundane and uninspiring work, are financially stressed, never go outdoors, skip meals, and eat an inadequate amount of calories.

Because constantly spending time trying to figure out what you should and shouldn't eat, and reading health books and blogs for hours a day is such a brain-tangling ███████, I like to see people pick other health battles than even think about what they are eating.

But back to healthy eating specifically. There are bigger things at play here.

It's extremely hard to figure out whether or not something is good or bad for you based on purely intellectual reasoning. Think coffee is bad for you? Well, there is a lot of good information about coffee being healthy. There is a lot of information and justification for it being unhealthy. I've been studying health and nutrition intensely for a decade, and you know what, I'm not sure if coffee is healthy or not. Or sugar. Or alcohol. Or chocolate. Or grains. Or legumes. Or meat. Or probiotics. Or vegetables. Or fruit. Or dairy.

I used to be able to give a definitive answer on each one of those things, but now I can't. I simply know too much to be sure, as there are numerous justifications for or against each one of the things I just listed. If you are sure about one of the above-listed things, that's because you've ingested one set of information and haven't investigated the other side of the story. If you had, you would be equally as unsure as I am.

And even with things that we can all intellectually agree is unhealthy, such as a meal at McDonald's, there will be literally thousands of people that read this book who are freezing cold, or haven't slept through the night in years, or who are suffering from anxiety, yada yada. And most of those health-conscious people wouldn't DARE eat at McDonald's. But, to their surprise, they might find almost immediate relief from their health condition(s) if they were to go pig out on 2-3 double Cheeseburgers, an apple pie or two, and an ice cold Coke from none other than the infamous Mickey D's. Why? Because the calorie-density, digestibility, and salt and sugar-heavy load of a McDonald's meal is unparalleled. And for someone in a really low metabolic state, this can literally be the most therapeutic of all combinations. You might heal faster eating at McDonald's than trying to do it on organic, unrefined, wholesome, and nutritious food because such food is not as calorie-dense, has a higher water content, has more fiber, and is just too ████ filling and unexciting to foster the same level of calorie consumption.

So the unknowns about what is and isn't healthy for an individual at any given moment are so vast that they are beyond our ability to neatly file into categories of "good" and "bad."

I am quite serious about all this. I love the shocking but I'm truly not saying this for shock value. It would be easier to be liked and for this book to be well-received by continuing to re-affirm your beliefs about what is and isn't healthy, because when someone says something is healthy that you think isn't, you react with serious objection. And in this case, that objection is directed towards me. But my goal is not to be liked. My goal here is to provide accurate, truthful, and unbiased information based on my wealth of study and experience. Most of you reading this don't need to hear what is and isn't healthy based on macronutrient breakdowns, nutrient density, ratio of polysaccharides to monosaccharides, and fiber type and quantity. You need to move on from this overly analytical way of thinking. For health reasons.

Considering all of this, what is healthy eating?

Healthy eating, for a recovering chronic dieter, from a long-term sustainable standpoint once you've achieved the basic physiological competencies of healthy function (daily bowel movements without straining, normal body temperature, normal sex drive, ability to sleep through the night without waking, stable mood, steady energy levels, no major health problems, etc.), can be boiled down to just a few basic principles...

1. Eat complete "square" meals at regular mealtimes consistently, and include snacks if you get hungry or get cold in the hands and feet in between meals
2. Eat enough to feel full and satisfied but no more or no less

3. Eat the proportions of foods that feel most appealing at any given meal, such as salty foods, meats, broth/gelatin, dairy products, vegetables, sweet foods, raw foods, starches, etc.

4. Pay attention to basic biofeedback (body warmth/temperature in particular) to make minor changes in your daily eating habits and proportion of various types of foods

5. Eat predominantly nutritious foods as the base of your diet, with unlimited freedom to eat supplemental non-nutritive "junk" foods as desired

6. Drink fluids when thirsty, and to satisfy thirst (not to get warm, or take in more nutrients i.e. juicing, or any motivations other than thirst)

7. Eat a high ratio of saturated to polyunsaturated fats

Yes, #7 is the only remaining dietary minutiae that I've managed to hold onto all these years, as obesity-proneness, rate of cellular aging, cellular energy production, glucose metabolism, and metabolic rate are all very negatively influenced by consuming a great deal of polyunsaturated fat – linoleic acid and arachidonic acid specifically. This should come as no surprise as this is by far, by percentages, the biggest dietary change ever to take place in recent times – with a 1,450% increase of vegetable oil consumption in the 20th century in the United States for example, and very large increases in the intake of vegetable-oil derived products like margarine and shortening as well.

Vegetable oil from agricultural commodities like cottonseeds, corn, soy, canola, sunflower, safflower, grapeseeds, and others is where this tremendous leap in consumption comes from. The type of fat that predominates in these oils is linoleic acid (LA), a type of omega 6 polyunsaturated fat. If you've done even light reading on nutrition you will have certainly heard of the virtues of omega 3, a type of polyunsaturated fat with numerous health benefits attributed to it. The health attributes given to it stem from omega 3's ability to counteract the negative impact of LA and its end-product, Arachidonic Acid (AA). The answer is not so much to megadose on omega 3, which has negative consequences of its own, but to reduce the consumption of LA and AA.

When an excess of this type of fat is fed to pigs, chickens, and farm-raised fish, it dramatically increases the amount of AA and LA in the skin, fat, eggs (pig eggs?), and organs of those animals. This is where the large increase in dietary AA has come from in the past century in the modern diet.

Anyway, suffice it to say that this mass dietary change has been very biologically significant. It has changed the composition of human cells, tissues, breast milk, number and size of fat cells, metabolism, levels of inflammation, and more. It seems to be most effectively counteracted by the consumption of protective fats like coconut oil, cocoa butter (chocolate), and butterfat from dairy products, and yes of course butter itself. I don't mean to eat a high-fat diet (been there done that, still kinda tired). Just use these fats in place of the fats you normally use.

But I don't think there's a need to take this TOO seriously if you catch my drift. These fats are completely endemic to our modern food supply, and you would have to pretty severely hermitize yourself to avoid them – a much greater health and wellness liability than just letting go and eating whatever ▓▓▓ you want.

I simply recommend eating more fish, red meat, and dairy products over pork and poultry, and using coconut oil and real butter in your home kitchen instead of vegetable oils, fake butter, and Crisco. Maybe choose something besides deep-fried foods and stuff slathered in mayonnaise when you eat out at restaurants. I don't think this change has to be turned into a major life-suppressing diet. Just make some small, realistic, and sustainable changes here. I think you'll reap some long-term rewards by doing so or I wouldn't have taken the risk of sounding like a health guru to inform you about it. And no your cholesterol won't go up from this change and give you a heart attack. What are you reading health books from the 80's still? Still watching Richard Simmons on Betamax?

Now that we've gotten your WTF reaction to #7 out of the way, let's back up to the top of the healthy eating practices list…

1. Eat complete "square" meals at regular mealtimes consistently, and include snacks if you get hungry or cold in the hands and feet in between meals

Whether it's six meals a day or even one, regularity with your eating habits is a health asset. The body loves regularity and thrives off of it. While I wouldn't set an alarm to your mealtimes, it's a good habit to give food the attention it deserves. No matter what you are doing, working in regular mealtimes at relatively consistent times (within reason – I mean, go out and have dinner with your friends by all means) each day is important – especially for someone with a history of undereating. What I like best about this practice for someone with a history of overthinking food, is that it allows eating to become regimented and habitual. Eating on autopilot. This takes a lot of the stress and decision-making and neurotic fixation out of the equation.

So see what you can do to trim down the eating chaos. I personally wake up to a carb feast and my highest calorie meal of the day. Lunch is usually saltier and meatier than breakfast, with heavier, fattier foods. For dinner I eat something lighter such as a bowl of soup with toast or baked potato. Breakfast around 9am, lunch around 1pm, and dinner around 7pm. It's habitual enough to be almost completely effortless. Find a meal schedule that works for your body and your lifestyle and stick with it, taking "meal time" very seriously – not just skipping it because you're busy.

2. Eat enough to feel full and satisfied but no more or no less

As you'll see later, sometimes recovery requires eating a little more food than you are used to, until your metabolism rises. But after that, there's really no reason to eat any more or less than you want to eat. Complete diet recovery involves neutrality with food, and there's simply no reason to eat a single bite more or less than you care for. Your body guides your food intake and expenditure without any calculations or interference on your behalf. Just let it do what it is programmed to do and get ███ out of the way. You'll quickly find that your body does a much better job of managing things than your brain. If hungry, eat. If full, stop. Continue for rest of life.

3.   Eat the proportions of foods that feel most appealing at any given meal, such as salty foods, meats, broth/gelatin, dairy products, vegetables, sweet foods, raw foods, starches, etc.

The ultimate place to eat all your meals would be a buffet, with an endless spread of different tastes, smells, textures, flavors, and varieties. Then you would truly be able to navigate through and find exactly what's most appealing, letting your body's senses guide you towards what you really want to eat. This would give you an opportunity to truly eat what you want to eat, in the exact quantity for each food type that you desire. A buffet has a tremendous way of equaling the playing field and neutralizing your food fixations as well. When you have unlimited, unadulterated access to everything you could possibly want, all the time, consistently, you lose your obsessions with all foods very quickly. In other words, your appetite is regulated with your body's needs, without the interference of restriction or "the knowledge of good and evil" when it comes to food.

Plus, I find combining several components together and achieving meal completeness – with something salty, something meaty, something crunchy, something starchy, something hot, something cold, something sweet, something brothy… yields substantial improvements to metabolism, digestion, mood, and all things related to these vital systems. While we can't create a huge spread of different foods for ourselves for every meal from a practicality standpoint, at the very least I encourage you to incorporate several components at each meal, with a particular emphasis on sweet, salty, and starchy – the ultimate de-stressing metabolic fuels. Yes, I'm all about food-combining!

Combine as many foods together as possible! And purposefully seek out variety to keep your diet fresh, exciting, and new.

4. Pay attention to basic biofeedback (body warmth/temperature in particular) to make minor changes in your daily eating habits and proportion of various types of foods

Along the same lines, your desires for certain foods is only one form of feedback for deciding what you're going to eat, and how much of the relative proportions of different kinds of food you are going to eat. For example, a spicy, meaty, smoky chili full of beans is damn pleasing to my senses. But too many beans and my stomach just blows up like a balloon. So what sounds tasty is not the only factor involved in what I choose to eat. You may also notice that eating too much meat in proportion to carbohydrates makes your feet icy cold, or too much fruit in proportion to less watery foods. Let this biofeedback dictate the proportions that you eat of various things.

Just don't get too carried away with this. For starters it can turn very neurotic – there are many things that determine how you respond to a meal. Get a horrible night's sleep for example and you'll probably crash and be cold after breakfast no matter what you eat. If you are myopically focused on food you'll drive yourself nuts trying to figure out why your breakfast didn't "work." Secondly, biofeedback can be misleading. An anorexic will feel the best after not eating, or eating a low-carb or low-calorie meal so that the high adrenaline state is perpetuated. Eating causes a big crash in mood, temperatures, and more with digestive discomforts, breakouts, and every ill you can imagine. Some people need to eat in a way that makes them feel their absolute worst to heal. But ultimately your biofeedback should factor into your food choices when appropriate, but only you can decide that for yourself, and that's not always an easy decision to make.

5. Eat predominantly nutritious foods as the base of your diet, with unlimited freedom to eat supplemental non-nutritive "junk" foods as desired

If you are just coming off of a lifelong joyless eating regime you might, for a while, just want to go berserk eating the junkiest diet you can get your hands on. That's quite alright. You might not feel your best, but ultimately doing so will neutralize those foods you've demonized and allow you to choose healthier foods for no other reason than they taste better and you like how they make you feel – the essence of having achieved full diet recovery. I still recommend eating a lot of nutritious foods as a general rule. I make stews, and eat greens, and drink fruit juice, and eat lots of dairy products, tons of fruit, root vegetables, and meats – that kind of thing. We do need micronutrients. But there's no food so junky that I truly wouldn't "touch it with a 10-foot pole." This easygoing relationship with the modern food environment is a health asset, not a liability. Just think of nutritious foods as a foundation and junk as a supplement, and I think you'll be fine.

I would also encourage you to get real about what is and isn't nutritious. Ice cream has the same nutrient content as human breast milk almost exactly. Pizza is extraordinarily nutritious. It's almost a calcium overload. Cheeseburgers have lots of nutrients. I squeeze an egg and 2-ounces of milk into every slice of French toast I eat at home. You don't have to drink kale juice all day to get adequate nutrients, and if you did you would obliterate your thyroid gland (kale is a goitrogen). It's not all about nutrients people, and some nutrients, like iron, may do more harm than good depending on the person. So just eat. Don't worry about it so much. I truly don't think that the health problems people are suffering from in the modern world are from nutrient deficiency. And if you aren't dieting and keeping yourself in a better metabolic state, you use nutrients a LOT more efficiently. You certainly don't need a diet high in minerals to maintain strong bones and teeth or whatever you think you need all that "nutrition" for.

6. Drink fluids when thirsty, and to satisfy thirst (not to get warm, or take in more nutrients i.e. juicing, or any motivations other than thirst)

Last but not least on the list of healthy "eating" habits is to apply the same general principle to your fluid intake. We'll talk more about this later on, as it is surprisingly significant, particularly for your metabolic rate – enough to write a whole book about it (*Eat for Heat*). order!

Finding the right fluid intake – total of all beverages and fluids naturally found in food, is a matter of using a combination of biofeedback and natural cues (just like what and how much to eat). The biofeedback goal is to urinate about once every four hours while awake and none in the middle of the night, with a nice yellow color to it each time. Adjust fluid intake accordingly to meet those goals.

Our natural thirst is of course a big factor in determining how much to drink as well. If you are thirsty, you probably need to drink. If you are not thirsty, you probably don't. But we have a modern habit of compulsively sipping beverages all day long. Health nerds often have it worse because they are juicing, drinking magic teas, guzzling massive smoothies, and often eating food with a much higher water content on top of all that. Be careful, as the overconsumption of fluids to the point where your urine becomes clear activates the stress system (and causes body temperature to typically plummet), and a dry mouth is a common symptom when the stress system is activated. This is NOT genuine thirst, so we can't rely exclusively on our thirst mechanism to guide us.

But at the very least, do not drink a bunch of fluids when you are not thirsty, as it can trigger this downward spiral if you do. If you are peeing clear, in rapid succession, you probably need to EAT, not drink, and do so immediately.

So I guess this concludes the section on Healthy Eating. This is really meant to be a general guide on how to get your nose out of a book or computer screen in trying to determine what you should ingest, and instead reconnect with your body – both its cues for certain things and its reaction to them. But keep thinking well-beyond your diet when you think of your health and the quality of your life overall – something we'll discuss in greater detail before we wrap this up. Put your diet increasingly on autopilot with some of the simple methods above.

Let's take a break from this line of thinking and turn our attention towards how to assess your metabolism and what to do to rehabilitate it if needed.

Metabolism Assessment

How do you know whether your metabolism is good or bad? High or low?

Well I would certainly recommend thinking well beyond the thyroid gland. You can get your blood levels tested if you want, but you have all the tools and information to assess your total net metabolic drive without any tests. The tests themselves are also very misleading, sometimes showing perfectly normal thyroid hormone levels in someone with a 96-degree body temperature, chronic constipation, hair loss, and wicked cold hands and feet – even in hot temperatures.

If it feels like a low metabolism, smells like a low metabolism, talks like a low metabolism, and looks like a low metabolism – it's a low metabolism. There is a lot more involved in metabolic rate and health than just the thyroid hormones (such as leptin, cortisol, adrenaline), which is why thyroid hormone supplementation is usually so ineffective compared to what is achievable through the strategies we'll discuss here.

The most important outwardly indicator of whether your body is using energy at full capacity, or conserving energy and producing it poorly at the cellular level, is your body temperature. Body temperature, and overall feeling of body warmth is one of the first things to go when metabolism starts to drop. I would highly recommend getting familiar with your body temperature. If you are highly overweight you may feel quite warm with all those extra layers, but don't let that fool you. The thermometer will tell a different story, particularly first thing in the morning.

The best times to check temperature are:

1. First thing in the morning before you even get out of bed
2. Before and after meals to see if it is going up or down in response to food
3. Late afternoon/early evening

For testing I don't recommend anything fancy. Just a simple Vick's digital thermometer found in most supermarkets and drug stores is as good as any.

I can already see you turning this into an obsessive habit. Hey, I haven't checked my own body temperature IN OVER A YEAR. But if you don't know what your body temperature is, and you have some symptoms that suggest that your metabolism may be significantly reduced, get to know what your body temperature is. If it is noticeably low at one or more of the testing times listed above (below 98 degrees F on an oral or rectal reading at any time suggests a little metabolic mediocrity – lower temperatures are even more indicative), play around with some of the information in this book and see if you can bump it up. If the past experience of others holds true for you, you've got at least a 90% shot at increasing it significantly all on your own with no drug or supplement interventions.

I also encourage you to redirect your obsessive focus on the small and insignificant details of what you are eating, and pay a lot more attention to the warmth of your hands and feet. The warmth of the extremities tells us two things – either your blood volume is reduced, causing poor circulation (a sign of reduced metabolic rate), or your stress system is activated, which shuts down the blood vessels in your extremities and causes feet, hands, and the tip of your nose to get chilly. Neither is good, and both are associated with being an old fart with a horrendous metabolism. If you find that your hands and feet are icy cold a lot of the time, maybe even so cold they are discolored, this too is a very strong sign of having a reduced metabolic rate.

Here are some of the other most common signs that your metabolism is lower than what is considered optimal. You may have some of the signs but not others. I suggest taking a tally of as many things as possible when assessing whether your metabolism is great or totally blows. And no, being thin or fat has nothing to do with your metabolic rate per se. The lowest metabolic rates are typically found in the underweight, not the overweight. Likewise you can have accumulated some extra weight but currently be in a nearly flawless metabolic state. Weight is pretty irrelevant to the task at hand here. Anyway, you probably already have your suspicions after reading up to this point, but here are some of the most common things that people notice when metabolic rate is reduced (and notice improving when it comes up)…

- Thin outer-third of your eyebrows
- Dry, thin slow-growing hair (body hair and the hair on your head)
- Cracked, dry, slow-growing fingernails

- Inability to sleep through the night without waking up – wakeup usually 2-4am
- Slow moving bowels, with a tendency towards constipation
- Bloating after eating, with food sitting in your stomach like a rock
- Low sex drive, or sexual function (erectile dysfunction in men, vaginal dryness in women)
- Mood disorders like anxiety and depression
- Frequent urination
- Excessive thirst/dry mouth
- Brain fog, poor mental focus
- Lots of allergies and hypersensitivities
- Dry skin, particularly around the lower legs and hands
- No desire for physical activity/lethargy
- Falling or thinning hair, both hair on your head and body hair

Basically, you should feel like a sloth. But it may manifest in other ways. Virtually every system is linked to our rate of energy production at the cellular level. These just happen to be some of the most common things people experience.

You don't have to "diet" per se to achieve a low metabolic rate either. Stress is the cause of a decreased metabolic rate, and there are infinite causes of stress – dieting just happens to be one that has been a particular focus of mine since entering the twisted world of telling people what to eat.

Regardless of what your history is, or how you achieved a low metabolic rate (many people have a suppressed metabolic rate due to many hereditary, prenatal, and postnatal factors), it's still important that we all get on the same page here and define good, healthy function.

Basically, I want everyone to perform well on the following competencies. These competencies represent very basic systems of our bodies, and I find, as a health advisor to tens of thousands of people and coach to hundreds of individual clients, that when there is major improvement in some of these basic areas you often see a number of seemingly-unrelated health problems improve or go away altogether. The following are the areas I have chosen to focus on the most. Consider these a list of goals that any health interventions you pursue (or don't pursue) should catapult you towards. In other words, I like to see everyone...

1. Have a body temperature (oral, rectal, ear, forehead) at least above 98 degrees (36.7 C) all day long, with peaks after meals and in the late evening of over 99 (37.2 C). The ideal body temperature in my experience is around 99 degrees (37.2) all of the time, with peaks into the mid to high-99's (37.5 C), but that's the ideal. At the very least you should be over 98 all the time (36.7 C).

2. Have warm hands and feet the vast majority of the time. Of course, there are occasions when it is cold, you are walking barefoot on a tile floor, etc. where your feet just aren't going to be that warm. And few can truly keep their extremities warm ALL the time. But keeping them feeling warm (with blood flow, not 3 pairs of socks and UGGs!) most of the

time is a good benchmark for being in a high metabolism/low stress state.

3.   Have at least one major bowel movement, if not two or three, that is large, soft, and quickly-expelled with no straining whatsoever every day. Bowel transit time should be fast enough that bloating and gas production is fairly minimal – not enough time for food to ferment and putrefy in your system.

4.   Sleep soundly, with the ability to get 8 or more hours of uninterrupted sleep with NO WAKEUPS to pee or otherwise. The most common time for a wakeup is between 2-4 am when adrenaline is peaking. The lower the metabolic rate, the higher the adrenaline peak because metabolism and stress play a constant tug-of-war. If it gets high enough you wake up. If it gets worse beyond that you start having anxiety, heart palpitations, a racing mind, and inability to fall back asleep at all. So uninterrupted sleep can be a pretty good indicator of overall metabolism and should be everyone's goal to achieve. Plus, sleep is perhaps the ultimate pro-metabolic activity.

5.   Urinate once every 4 hours or so (roughly, set a timer to this and I kill you!) during the day and none at night. Each urination should have a consistent yellow or gold color to it (not clear, you'll notice body temperature often plummets when urine becomes clear). Each urination should also not be accompanied by a strong and sudden urge to urinate out of nowhere, making you feel like you need to

rush to the toilet to keep from wetting your pants (symptom of the stress response suddenly activating).

Nail the above and follow those changes where they lead. Spend enough time in that state, and health improvements in a number of areas is virtually guaranteed. Of course, there are many other competencies to focus on. Sex drive and function is a huge biomarker for a good metabolism. For women, a regular menstrual cycle with no PMS or cramps is another fantastic metabolism yardstick. Skin moisture, rate of fingernail and toenail growth, and rate of hair growth is another positive indicator. Strengthening teeth with less tooth sensitivity, even when eating sugary foods, is another positive indicator. I could list so many you would forget them all! Mark Starr's chapter on low-metabolism symptoms is 85 pages long!

Each area alone is not enough, but lump many different bodily systems and markers together and you can easily track progress with confidence.

Now let's talk about a multi-faceted approach to achieving these sweeping changes.

Rest and Refeeding

For most people, even those who are skeletal from a severe eating disorder, the recipe for rehabilitating metabolic rate, and even surpassing what is historically normal for you, is simply rest and food. Lots of both. Surplus is a good word. I wish the formula were more complicated and exotic so you could have more faith that it would do something magical. But, unfortunately, many of the answers to the seemingly-complex and obscure medical diagnoses are head-slappingly simple. Not all of course. I don't proclaim that you can expect to walk on water, or that food and rest will be enough for everyone. But it's all that's required for a lot of people to make significant progress. Progress is another good word. Chase that, not perfection or some utopian health state or else you will be sorely disappointed with this and every other health book, protocol, program, and health elixir you come across.

How much rest? Well, as much as you can reasonably get without getting fired from your job. By rest I mean primarily sleep, but generally taking it easy when you are awake is a great asset too. I wouldn't go so far as to recommend bed rest, as that will make you go stir-crazy, but you certainly would hinder and retard (the Alan Garner… *The Hangover*, pronunciation) the recovery process by working long hours in a frantic environment, doing a lot of hard (or even easy) exercise, or otherwise placing a high load of stress upon your system.

I emphasize the word "surplus" again. I wouldn't just recommend getting some good sleep at first, but getting an abnormal amount of sleep. 10 hours will heal you much more quickly than 8. Naps are great too unless you find them impairing your sleep at night.

It should really feel like you are giving yourself a spa vacation. Yeah, I know not everyone will be able to work that into their lives. Between kids, work, and the hustle and bustle of life that won't be practical. But it's good to at least identify what would be ideal with the goal of metabolic rehab in mind. Even little things like a 5-minute break to just relax and clear your mind is something, and might be more significant than you think it would be.

Other ways that you can achieve this "spa vacation" lifestyle during the healing process are encouraged. Massages, calming music, meditation, light stretching, warm baths, sunbathing, curious walks in a serene outdoor setting, relaxed breathing, raging fires in your fireplace, lounging around in comfortable clothes, snuggling, laying down and resting when you get the chance, reading something (besides health and nutrition books) – whatever sounds like it would make your whole body relax and enter that state where your eyes are heavy and mind is calm is great.

I'll let you figure out what you can and can't do, what is and isn't practical, what is and isn't relaxing, and so forth. The most important thing is perhaps the mindset of self-nurture, and completely abandoning the idea that you must do something productive or strenuous, or perk yourself up if you are feeling like doing absolutely nothing. You don't need more motivational speeches from your consciousness. You should enter a state of demotivation and really take it easy on yourself in whatever little ways you can. It's okay to rest. It's okay to be a slug. You have plenty of time in the future to kick ▓▓ and take names physically, mentally, and vocationally – doing so in a healthy state instead of one that is starved, stressed, strained, and sickly.

Don't get too discouraged or feel like you can't make progress if you can't spend your day getting massaged, sleeping 10 hours a day, and birdwatching in the park either. You can still heal with 6 kids running ▓▓▓▓▓ and no trust-fund or tit-warblers in sight. It just might take a little extra time and focus.

As far as what to do on the refeeding front, I'll go into more detail…

My original work was highly influenced by a religious faith in nutritious, unrefined, wholesome foods as the be-all, end-all of health. I don't have any problem with eating such things, but over the years I have found that soul-satisfying, liberating, and maximally-palatable foods enjoyed in an almost sensual way without guilt or much thought at all beyond "damn this Tiramisu is freaking awesome" work better. They work better for raising the metabolism, they work better for stifling stress, and they also go much farther in repairing your relationship with food and yourself. Just eat the food… whatever sounds good, with more focus on the sensory experience of luscious tastes and textures and less nutri-intellectualism providing a background of chatter over the health virtues or lack thereof of what you are ingesting.

In perhaps an ironic way, the lower your metabolic rate, the more therapeutic the "junk" foods really are. What people consider to be pleasure foods are things rich in fat and carbohydrates in a very soft, digestible, refined, and calorie-dense package with a low water content. We'll talk more about the significance of those qualities later. And, as you heal with foods that wouldn't appear on any health guru's list of approved foods, you later graduate to eating a diet much closer to what is considered to be the quintessential "healthy diet." And you won't gravitate to a healthy diet through iron will or anything like that either. You'll just come to prefer eating less calorie-dense foods once your body no longer needs a surplus of calories to do its repair work.

Now some specifics, so that you aren't left feeling totally unguided as to what to eat. I don't want to tell anyone what to eat, and want to empower you as much as possible to make your own choices. But for someone used to eating a Spartan health food diet this directionless approach is often a cause for anxiety and confusion, not liberation. So here we go…

Nothing I say beyond this point should be looked at as a verbatim prescription. I encourage you to take as many liberties as you want, even going so far as to challenge your food demons head on by eating them with courage and resilience. The following guidelines and specific foods mentioned are meant to be a conceptual aid, to sort of grasp what a metabolism-stoking diet might *kind of* look like – tailored to your own preferences (taste preferences rather than preferences arrived at from having health information diarrhea splattered all over your brain).

Now, follow these general guidelines…

1.   Wake up and eat some rapidly-absorbed carbohydrates as quickly as possible. Something like a pastry or toast smeared with salted butter and jam with a little fruit juice or sweetened whole milk – or weak coffee brewed in whole milk with lots of added sugar. The morning is the typical human peak in cortisol – the primary stress hormone. Getting carbohydrates into the system quickly starts to bring this hormone back down during this pivotal time. Remember, you haven't eaten in a long time, which in and of itself can be very stressful for someone with a reduced metabolic rate. Generally the stronger the metabolic rate the longer you can afford to go without food. The crappier your metabolism, the more frequently you need to eat.

I treat this period almost exactly how the mainstream nutrition world treats the post-workout period, as, hormonally, it's very similar. Stress hormones are peaking, body is depleted of glucose, etc. The faster you can shut that down the better, which is why post-workout formulas contain maltodextrin, waxy maize, dextrose, and similar substances with the highest known glycemic indexes. Fast-absorbing starch (bread, pancakes, tortillas, breakfast cereal, hash browns, homefries – something like that) with something sweet (sugar, jam, syrup, fruit, fruit juice) along with it is a great combination to achieve that objective.

2.   While it's still morning time, consume a more substantial and hearty breakfast, but still emphasize carbohydrates strongly. Really connect with what sounds the best at this time. It may be chocolate chip pancakes and pastries or French toast with fruit and juice. Or it may be something like steak and eggs and a glass of milk. Or it may be something off-the-wall like ice cream with chocolate sauce and a hot dog. You'll have to figure that out for yourself. But choose freely and keep it very calorie-dense and warming. We'll discuss how to structure your meals to give them a net-warming effect later (you can eat 2000 calories of oranges for breakfast but you would be freezing your ass off after, for reasons we'll delve into). Eat to absolute, can't eat another bite fullness if at all possible (I know not everyone's schedule accommodates morning feasting, and yes, I know I'm using parentheses excessively. Back off man).

The purpose of all the morning gorging is to get warm as early in the day as possible. The vast majority of people (not all) see the lowest body temperatures, and have the coldest hands and feet, during the first few hours of the day – with a particular tendency to crash out and feel icy cold mid-morning. Loading up on calories early is a great way to catapult you into a much higher metabolic state during the low point. Staying warm once you've gotten warm is a lot easier than the initial shove required to get temps over 98F.

3.   Eat regular, warming meals at regular meal times for the remainder of the day, putting a big emphasis on what I call the anti-stress s's – salt, sugar, and

starch. This is the Holy trinity of foods that you should try to combine as religiously as you can. To that you can add some saturated fat. Fat is necessary in my experience because it adds calorie density to the food and makes it much tastier, both qualities that lend to higher calorie consumption. It is the calories, after all, that bring the metabolism up.

4. By regular meals, I mean creating consistent mealtimes to the best of your ability and sticking with that. Food deserves enough of your attention that you stop whatever you are doing at least a couple times per day to eat – not when it's convenient, but when it's mealtime. The easiest template is to just create regular breakfast, lunch, and dinner times and try to stick to them. Regular rhythms are a big asset for someone carrying his or her metabolism up from the basement. For you, that might be a toast and jam eye-opener at 7, breakfast at 8, lunch at 1, and dinner at 7. All I ask is that you, at the very least, don't skip mealtimes altogether. A healthy person can get away with it. You, however, may not have graduated to that level yet.

5. Eat snacks whenever hands and feet are cold. Because the ability to go long periods without food and not see a significant drop in metabolism is typically compromised in someone in need of diet recovery, snacks are great. Meals, if they are big and tasty enough, should get you feeling warm. But this warmth may be fleeting. An hour or two after a meal you may notice that warmth going away and the hands and feet feeling chilly once more. Have a

snack, preferably something that combines the anti-stress S's – salt, sugar, and starch. Something like a handful of pretzels and some raisins. A couple of dates with a slice of cheese. Cheese and crackers with a few sips of a soft drink. Popcorn or chips and a few apple slices. That's all it really takes. Even if it doesn't warm your hands and feet up, at least know that you are still lowering your exposure to stress somewhat.

Other cues to be even more vigilant about these snacks would be other major signs of your stress system becoming active, such as blurred vision, mood changes, dizziness, a strong, sudden urge to urinate, frequent urination, dry mouth, and anything else you've noticed happening to you when you've gone too long without food in the past.

6. Do not take in too many fluids. This includes all fluids found in food and beverages. An apple, for example, is not a drink, but it contains fluid just the same as a glass of water. Excess fluid is the nemesis (downfall) of body temperature, which is one reason that calorie-dense foods that few would consider "health food" are great for metabolic rehab. As metabolism rises, the need for fluids as well as your ability to handle them without flooring your metabolic rate increases.

It's best, at first, to drink based more on how frequently you urinate and what the color of that urine is. Aim for urinating once every four hours during the day and none during the night, always with some nice yellow color to it. Increase your ratio of calories and salt to fluids in order to achieve this at first. But after you've gotten out of the initial metabolic hole, it's best to then turn to drinking based more on thirst cues, as you will start getting really thirsty as that body temperature comes up. Obey the high metabolism thirst, or else you are likely to start having problems like restless legs and severe headaches in the late afternoon and early evening.

We'll discuss this more in the next chapter, as this concept can be a little confusing, but it's very important that you get it. It makes this process a lot more efficient, expedient, and precise. I am actually including a full chapter from my book *Eat for Heat,* which discusses the role of fluid balance in metabolism exhaustively to help you fully get it.

Those are the basics in terms of how to go about raising metabolic rate on the food end. Not exotic no. No need for Amazonian Acai-fed fermented piranha eggs or other superfoods. And in actuality, you can still make great headway with your metabolic rate without even paying a whole lot of attention to the above details. If you were to just put this book down right now and work on getting more sleep, de-stressing, taking a break from hard exercise, and just eat as much of whatever sounds most delicious as you desire every time you feel like there's room in your stomach, you would still pull it off.

The last bit of advice I have for you is quite basic and should be implied from what we've covered already, but it needs to be said as plainly and clearly as possible – *eat plenty of everything.* When I first started developing a protocol for raising metabolism with all those fancy bullet-points n' everything, we (me and my most vocal participants) started referring to the protocol as "The High Everything Diet (HED)." Yeah, names are fun and acronyms are even better. I mean, there's a real shortage of acronyms out there. I have felt compelled over the years to add to the pool.

But the HED was as the name implies, high in everything. In a world obsessed with low-calorie, low-carb, low-fat, low-this, and low-that – the concept here was pretty obvious. Don't restrict anything. Eat it all. Eat all the carbs, fat, and protein you want. Sure, you'll have your favorites and tilt the balance a little one way or another (I recommend tilting it towards carbs if possible, but I think, really, that what's most therapeutic is tilting it in the other direction in relation to where you have been on your most recent diet escapades), but don't limit or restrict.

Eat salt. And sweets. And meats. And veggies. Root vegetables. Grains. Dairy products. Eat all the things you could ever want. Fill all those tanks, especially the ones that you have left empty in your dieting career.

And most of all, eat a lot of calories. Some people I'm discovering, still don't succeed when they just eat as much as they want, or even eat a little bit more than they want. With a really low metabolism, and with a history of eating disorders, calorieality is often skewed.

This process is all about surplus calories for repair work. Gwyneth Olwyn of www.youreatopia.com, a site specializing in recovering from restrictive eating patterns of varying degrees of severity, summed it up well…

"Recovery is the opposite process of dieting. With dieting you create a calorie deficit so that your body makes up the difference by using energy stores in fat, bone, muscles and major organs. But with recovery, you have to provide not only enough energy to replenish fat tissue, but also even more energy is required to reverse pervasive physiological damage.

"When you dependably eat the minimum calories every day (often much more than that when you feel like it), you won't get stuck in a quasi-recovered state that usually leads to relapse or a shift from frank anorexia to restrict/reactive eating cycles."

So, while I hate throwing around numbers when I really want to see everyone ceasing to count calories, carbs, or even really thinking about what or how much they are eating to achieve full recovery, in the beginning numbers can serve a purpose.

Everyone has their own way of calculating calorie requirements. The main thing to insure success with the objective we're after is making sure that we overshoot your basic needs to achieve metabolism-stimulating surplus. Here's what I have found based on the food reports of others, my own experience, and the common calculations that I've seen used elsewhere…

Because everyone has varying levels of muscle mass, it's best for everyone, as a baseline, to estimate their body weight with very little fat on it. This obviously cannot be precise, but most people have a decent idea of what they feel is their ideal body weight (although when you add a lot of bone mass, muscle mass, organ mass and more during this process you may find you look great, even better than ever before and leaner too at a much higher weight than you expected).

Take this hypothetical, estimated ideal body composition in pounds – let's call it 150 pounds since that is average, and multiply it by 20 if you are a woman and 23 if you are a man.

$$150*20 = 3000$$
$$150*23 = 3450$$

The reason for the difference is that a reasonably lean man and a reasonably lean woman have different body compositions. A man should have more muscle mass and less body fat, and thus have slightly higher metabolic needs than a woman even if scale weight is exactly the same. But, truth be told – and most people know this intuitively, women have higher metabolic rates than men on a lean body weight-adjusted scale. Face it, they are way hotter. No, actually they are. Women tend to have higher peak body temperatures than men – typically coinciding with ovulation and entry to the 2nd half of the menstrual cycle. I actually created a "hot chicks club" for women over 99 degrees F. And, I will add, most women I know can eat just as much as I can despite having way less lean tissue than I have, and my metabolism, while not superhuman, certainly isn't low.

Anyway, those calculations should serve as THE ABSOLUTE MINIMUM amount of calories one should consume on the journey from low metabolic rate to high metabolic rate. With tasty food, it ain't hard. And I wouldn't necessarily back off the calories when body temperature gets up. Rather, I like to see people work on strength and fitness levels while continuing to eat beyond their basal needs.

If you are consuming way more calories than that, great. It's natural if you are coming out of a dieted state to see a rapid surge in appetite as you begin refeeding. That big appetite begins to taper as body temperature normalizes. And if it doesn't, that's fine too. The body manages surplus calories very well, increasing the amount passed in stool, increasing physical energy and fidgeting, increasing body heat, and increasing the desire and threshold for exercise. Some people report eating over 8,000 calories per day consistently, without gaining weight, and without going out of their way to forcefully burn calories.

Even a 120-pound woman wrote in the week I'm writing this very paragraph about consistently eating 3500-5000 calories per day and maintaining a rock solid 120 pound bodyweight with no fluctuations.

And yes, if you are over age 30, you will probably consume fewer calories because your metabolism isn't as high as it is in youth, and there is a decline in metabolism with aging that is probably not overturnable (not actually a word, but I think it works). Make sure to eat enough to get that temperature up. Don't be overwhelmed or daunted by the task of eating 4000+ calories per day. Odds are you will have success with far fewer. But don't be too much of a little bitch about it and think you're too old for this or that this program doesn't work for post-menopausal women and their "unique hormonal needs." Still eat that food. If you must calculate, use the formulas above but subtract 1% for every year in age over 30. At age 60 let's say, the above formula might be downgraded by 30%. (60-30=30).

The only other thing you might want to give a number to is carbs, especially if you have been a habitual carbophobe for many years. To determine MINIMUM carbohydrate levels, take your minimum calorie levels calculated above, and divide that number by 8.

For me that's…

$$200*23 = 4600$$
$$4600/8 = \underline{575}$$

That 575 is the minimal number of grams of carbohydrates per day needed for optimal recovery, and is equal to about 50% of total caloric intake. But like I said, I would rather see most people slightly tilted to the high-carb side for recovery because of the superior properties of sugar and starch for metabolic recovery. 60% carbs might be even better than just half of your energy coming from carbohydrates. Much higher than that though and food becomes too unenjoyable to pack in adequate calories, in my experience. Although you are more than welcome to try it.

As a final word to this chapter specific to refeeding, if your metabolism is pretty strong, you don't display many of the signs and symptoms of a low metabolism, your body temperature is normal or close to it – it's probably not a good idea to purposefully and forcefully raise your calorie intake really high. Going through a refeeding phase is extremely therapeutic to those who need it, but not everyone does. I don't think it will harm anyone to spike their calories a little bit, getting in a surplus, but don't take a "medicine" that you don't need.

If you don't really need refeeding, don't do it. Just eat well, avoid skipping too many meals or going on some diets with a naïve belief that this will make you lean long-term. Eat to appetite when you are hungry but not beyond, be consistent, make time in your day for eating – the basics. You get what I'm saying here. I hope.

Perfecting Fluid Intake

We live in a world where everyone from your doctor to the local nutritionist to the athlete believes that plain water should be consumed in large amounts every day. While really healthy people can get away with taking in fluids beyond physiological needs, general prescriptions to drink 8-8-ounces glasses of water per day is very detrimental and even dangerous for someone with a very suppressed metabolism.

When metabolic rate is low, fluid needs decrease. If you have lost a bunch of weight with a diet, your fluid needs decrease in proportion to your loss of size. But more important than all of that – when metabolism is low your body wastes salt. And what's called "osmoregulation," or your body's ability to manage levels of electrolytes in your fluids becomes significantly impaired as well.

What does all this mean?

It adds up to making sure you are taking in the right amount of fluids, because if you drink too much you run the risk of experiencing some very pronounced symptoms from having body fluids that are too diluted – watered down. This watered down state is known formally as "hyponatremia," or having too much water in proportion to sodium in your blood. But blood is just one place this shows up. I commonly see people displaying many mild symptoms of hyponatremia all the time, with or without blood tests to confirm this. These symptoms often overlap with the symptoms of hypoglycemia, and I actually think hyponatremia, or low salt levels, is much more common than having low glucose levels.

Here are some common symptoms of hyponatremia. Keep in mind that if you are peeing clear, urinating frequently, peeing all night, and suffering from what otherwise are extremely common low metabolism symptoms – that this very diluted urine represents all of your extracellular fluid, including your blood, being very watered down…

From the Mayo Clinic, some symptoms of hyponatremia include…

- Nausea and vomiting
- Headache
- Confusion
- Loss of energy
- Fatigue
- Restlessness and irritability
- Muscle weakness, spasms or cramps
- Seizures

To that you can add many other symptoms synonymous with hyponatremia or water intoxication as it is also known, such as blurred vision, frequent urination, migraines, extremely cold hands and feet, anxiety, rapid or erratic pulse, and more.

Perfecting fluid intake isn't something you do based on any chart or equation. There is no place I can direct you for calculating this. Rather, like I mentioned already (like 3 times to make sure you don't forget it), you should take in the amount of fluids that results in you urinating roughly once every four hours – always with some good yellow color to it.

Yes I know you've heard you should drink a ton of water, and that your urine should be clear. This is one of the greatest health travesties to befall the general public. If urine concentration falls below a certain level in a pet or horse or something, veterinarians take this very seriously and assume something is really wrong with the animal. Yet in humans we are actually striving for this, and it takes a toll – manifesting in a reduced body temperature, and all that tends to come with it.

Of course, it's not just water found in a bottle or glass that you have to worry about. Water is found in everything – from salad to tea, from pepperoni pizza to watermelon. Excess water from any source is anti-metabolic, and drinking too much can literally prevent you from fully recovering and reaching a normal or above-normal core temperature.

Because of this, I think it's worth it to make you a little more conscientious, especially those of you in need of serious recovery (maybe you are trying to recover from a full-blown eating disorder or something), about the total number of calories you are eating in proportion to the total fluid content. Generally, a higher ratio of calories to water content, the more metabolically-stimulating that food is.

Take ice cream for example. It's got about 1,000 calories per pint. Skim milk has 1,000 calories per 3 quarts/liters. If you eat 1,000 calories of ice cream your core temperature will should rise and you'll feel warmer. If you drink 1,000 calories of skim milk it will leave you freezing cold, and you'll see your core temperature probably drop substantially – coinciding with cold hands and feet, feeling pretty awful and maybe even showing some serious symptoms of hyponatremia, and of course, urinating frequently with totally clear urine.

That's why I say that more concentrated and calorie-dense foods usually work a lot better for someone in an impaired metabolic state. I'm certainly an advocate for nutritious food consumption, but that is an afterthought compared to the much greater priority of getting metabolism normalized. And to do that, you simply must eat calorie-dense foods that have, by definition, a high ratio of calories to water content. You cannot heal your metabolism on a diet of watermelon, vegetables, and skim milk. The more of those you consume, the colder and more dangerously ill you are likely to become.

I wrote an entire book about this simple principle in *Eat for Heat: The Metabolic Approach to Food and Drink*, which is a fantastic companion to this book. But because few will read both, I thought it worthy to at least include a big portion of one important conceptual chapter from it – the chapter on "Warming Food vs. Cooling Food." This chapter will help you to structure your meals and snacks in such a way as to achieve the net-warming effect from food – getting those hands and feet warm and body temperature significantly higher immediately. It also contains some much needed discussion on beverages, which we have yet to spend much time discussing…

Warming Food, Cooling Food

...So one thing I often say is...

"You can eat a whole entire pizza, but if you drink a gallon of water with it you're likely to be freezing cold and peeing your brains out an hour later. Eat a single slice of pizza but only have a couple sips of a beverage with it and you'll be warm and toasty later."

You can see the basic concept at play here, and you can experiment with this a little bit yourself to validate it if you want. The guiding idea is manipulating the ratio of food to fluids. I think when you start tinkle tinkering it will become obvious.

Likewise, I also often mention something like...

"If you wake up and eat a bowl of watery oatmeal for breakfast with a glass of milk and 3 big slices of watermelon you'll be peeing and freezing all morning."

This is, of course, because the water content is so high – especially in proportion to the amount of salt in a breakfast like that.

Or...

"It doesn't matter how much watermelon you eat, it will never make you warm. The amount of calories and sodium in proportion to the water content makes it impossible."

So anyway, what I'm getting at is that some foods are warming. Some are cooling. Drinks of all kinds are generally cooling unless it is extremely calorie dense, like half and half with molasses added ("halfasses" I call it – yes it's better than it sounds, and yes I am hilarious thank you for noticing).

The beauty of this revelation, I think, is being able to achieve the net-warming effect of eating – something that is not an easy task for someone with a suppressed metabolic rate, and keep the stress system suppressed and the metabolism high. Well, not only that you can achieve that, but that you can do it without necessarily blatantly overconsuming food to the point of being stuffed – a tactic that I relied on exclusively before coming across this increasingly precise way to do business (you should still eat to fullness though, no matter what).

The most warming substances, in my experience, are sugar, starch, and salt – with saturated fat as an honorable mention. Well, any fat is warming because of the calorie-density of fat, but dairy, red meat, cocoa, and coconut fats (the most saturated sources) theoretically should have the best long-term preservation of metabolism and mitochondrial energy production. Thus was born the...

"Anti-Stress S's" – sugar, starch, salt, and saturated fat.

And that's just in terms of food. Other anti-stress S's include sleep, sun, saltwater (as in hanging out on the beach, but may also include salt-water baths and the actual salty water itself), and perhaps sex (although that depends on the context).

None of these really work in isolation, not even the salt – as we need carbohydrates to actually assimilate the salt, which is why rehydration drinks contain both salts/electrolytes and glucose. I find they work best when combined together. They taste better combined together too – all the edible S's that is, which fosters greater calorie consumption and subsequently obtaining the necessary amount of calories required to obtain or maintain a healthy metabolism.

Not everyone has universally noticed the warming effects of any one type of food as was revealed in a survey-esque article I wrote entitled "What Gets You Hot?" But generally the yummy foods, and yummy meals get it done the best. You'll note that meals that include a combination of several of the items below have the greatest warming effect.

Some of the superstars are:

• Cheese – with the high calorie density, high salt content, and extremely low water content it's hard to go wrong with cheese, or things that have lots of cheese on them like pizza, grilled cheese sandwiches, or cheeseburgers

• Coconut – Coconut oil is renowned for its ability to assist with metabolic rate and body heat, but any source of coconut will do. The medium-chain saturated fatty acids seem to be the active warming ingredient. Coconut is of course very calorie dense with a low water content, and cooking foods in oil of any kind increases the calorie to water ratio

• Chocolate – Calorie dense with a low water content and some sugar in it too. I can't overdo it on the chocolate or my bed sheets get drenched with sweat

• Flours – Flours made from grains, wheat of course being the most common, have very high calorie density and no water content at all until some liquid is added in the preparation of things like bread, crackers, pastries, tortillas, cookies, and so on. With the high starch levels and calorie density, and their palatability, flour-products are generally very warming

• Red Meat – It's not always warming, but generally the fattier cuts of red meat like beef and lamb are very warming. Fatty red meat is very calorie dense, and it also absorbs a phenomenal amount of salt before it becomes disgustingly salty. A double cheeseburger at Mickey D's has more salt than an entire large bag of Sea Salt Kettle Chips, yet the chips actually taste saltier

• Potatoes – Potatoes are not as calorie dense as other foods, but with their high starch levels and the large quantity of salt they require to be maximally palatable, potatoes fried in coconut oil or mashed with butter are an old warming standby in my house. All varieties of sweet potatoes and yams are great too, as are the less commonly used tubers like yucca and taro

• Soy sauce – Soy sauce is very warming due to its extreme saltiness, and the taste is outstanding, which fosters a total salt consumption that is much higher than when you use regular table salt to season your food

• Ice cream – Ice cream packs quite a lot of energy per unit of volume, and lots of sugar without the high water content of fruit or juice. It's cold, but most feel very warm after eating some ice cream and similar desserts like cheesecake, panna cotta, or pudding

• Other desserts – Any of the typical dessert-type foods, including cookies, pastries, pies, cakes, and just about anything you can think of are extremely warming due to the palatability, low water content, and high sugar content of most desserts

Now on to the cooling foods/substances...

• Water – Of course. The only time water seems to have a warming effect is when you are truly dehydrated and your stress system is activated by it. Otherwise it is generally cooling

• Coffee and tea – I don't think these are exceptionally cooling, but tend to have a cooling effect because people consume them when they are cold and are hoping to warm up. In the short-term the temperature of them is warming, but it perpetuates the coldness. The lower the metabolic rate, the higher the desire to drink warm fluids and to take in stimulants, so one should really use caution when it comes to consuming coffee and tea regularly

• Soft Drinks – Soft drinks are generally considered to be the single most fattening substance in the modern diet. That's a bold proclamation, as no food or drink in isolation is truly inherently fattening. But soft drinks do encourage drinking beyond thirst, drinking beyond thirst does lower body temperature (which reduces metabolic rate and calorie burn at rest by a substantial amount), and anything that lowers calorie burn while providing a lot of calories to go with it is a prime suspect in the separation in equality between calories burned and calories consumed that leads to changes in body weight

• Juice – Juice shares many similarities to soft drinks and in my experience is even more cooling than soft drinks, perhaps due to the high potassium content of most juices

• Diet Drinks – Diet drinks are the granddaddy of them all. Sweeteners like aspartame are extremely sweet and also cause excitation in the brain. Throw in some caffeine and you've got something very attractive. I notice that it's very common for diet drink consumers to consume outrageous quantities, and diet drink consumption has been tied to many symptoms indistinguishable from the symptoms of excess water consumption – like headaches, migraines, and seizures. Diet drinks are worse because they provide no sugar, unlike juice and sugared soft drinks. The cooling effect is similar to water, but the qualities of diet drinks foster much greater consumption beyond physiological need

• Lowfat Milk – Eat a few bowls of cereal (who eats just one?) with whole milk – you might be warm. Eat a few bowls of cereal with skim milk and forget about it. The removal of saturated fats and most of the calories seems to make milk function less like a meal, and more like a glass of water consumed beyond physiological fluid needs

• Soup – Soup is warming short-term because of the temperature. But soup can be cooling too. It's very filling. To actually get enough calories from most soups you would have to consume far too much fluid. But soups like the potato soup I make, cooked in whole milk, with lots of added salt, butter, and cheese is actually warming. But those things have to be added to keep it from being cooling. The same could be said for oatmeal and other porridges

•Fruit – Fruit, with its high water content, low calorie-density, and high potassium to sodium ratio is amongst the most cooling of all foods. A little is fine. Going beyond physiological fluid needs with fruit is extremely cooling. Same could be said of smoothies, especially ones made with just frozen fruit and juice, or lowfat yoghurt or soy milk or something. Brrrr. Would be nice in the tropics and in the summer when it's actually advantageous to be cooler though. Adding salt to fruit, as is done where I grew up with things like citrus and watermelon, helps a lot. But that can be said of any of the things listed on this page

•Vegetables – Like fruit, vegetables can be very cooling for the same reasons. Few people overconsume vegetables, but it can be done, especially if you are doing a lot of juicing

These are decent lists to start with, but even so, looking at these lists doesn't really tell the whole story of what I'm trying to convey. Not at all really, because no one just sits down and eats nothing but fruit. Well, some do. But anyone remotely in tune with their body's needs, cravings, and biofeedback will have gotten past such a phase hopefully.

This list is in no way an attempt to steer you towards the warming list at the exclusion of the cooling list. If you do that you'll croak. You can't just eat pizza and cookies and chug a glass of soy sauce and not take any complementary fluids with it. The higher your metabolic rate, and if you do any strenuous exercise (which you probably should once your health is fairly stable), the more fluids and thus cooling foods you will need to consume.

Now don't freak out on me because all the foods on the warming list are "bad" for you. Such foods can be taken to excess no doubt, but such foods are incredibly therapeutic for the journey from having a low metabolism to a normal or above-normal metabolic rate. The irony is that if you are in rough metabolic shape – let's say you have dieted extensively, you will actually need to eat "unhealthy" food for a while in order to graduate to eating a "healthy diet." I know that sounds weird, but try dieting. Does it increase or decrease your cravings for the items on list 1 or list 2? I rest my case. And this is actually a beautiful thing that your body does to save you from yourself. Binging on junk food is actually what your body does to heal itself from the harms various forms of self-deprecating eating and exercise programs deliver.

I can still hear you going off on a tangent about the stuff you've read about fructose, the processing of table salt, the glutamic acid in soy sauce, the hormones in ice cream, the evil villainous gluten, the lack of vitamins or fiber in white flour, or otherwise. As someone who spent the better part of a decade wrapped up in such relative minutiae, I highly encourage you to let go of a lot of that fluff and give this a try. Your fears and the things you are ideologically tethered to from excess internet health reading will hopefully fade pretty quickly until you are eating a more sustainable and socially-reasonable diet, and feeling a heck of a lot better than you were when intellectualizing every last detail of your food choices.

If you're not hip to that, that's fine too. As Uncle Rico said in Napolean Dynamite, "Stop wishing, and call me when you're ready ."

But regardless of what you believe, and what you feel is appropriate and "safe" for you to eat personally, you can still of course apply the basic principles we're discussing here. You can eat all the grassfed yak butter and goji juice and Himalayan beetle pus and tree bark that you want. Just put some soy sauce on it and stop drinking so much ▆▆▆ water.

What I meant by putting together these lists are to help you become aware of the connections, and learn to balance things appropriately. Here are some examples of how you might actually think about things as you go to construct a meal...

If you are going to eat oatmeal for example, that's absolutely fine. But if you eat it plain, cooked in water with no salt added, it will tank your metabolism. Try cooking it in milk and adding sugar, salt, and butter. Problem solved. Net effect: warming.

Likewise, if you are going to eat oatmeal for breakfast, don't make it too watery like soup. Also take note of the fact that there is a lot of fluid in the oatmeal. Oatmeal is a water-rich food. You wouldn't want to complement the meal with other water-rich things like a big glass of milk and 2 oranges, or a smoothie let's say. You might be better off complementing it with something very salty with a low water content, like a couple slices of cheese and only a small handful of fruit – added to the oatmeal perhaps. That would be a great warming meal, and be complete with sufficient calories and the full constellation of S foods – sugar, starch, salt, and saturated fat. This same line of thinking can be applied to all kinds of porridges, breakfast cereal with milk (don't drown it!), soups, etc.

Or let's say that you really feel that fruit is a healthy food for you, and you like it. Well, that may or may not be true depending on who you are and what kind of metabolic state you're in. The main thing is that you don't wash your metabolism out and activate your stress system. You could sprinkle some salt on it, or let it marinate in a pinch of salt. Trust me, some strawberries or peaches marinated in a little salt won't hurt the flavor.

Or you could do the same with sugar – put a little sugar or maple syrup over the fruit and let it marinate for a little bit.

Or you could have a fingerlickin' grilled cheese sandwich laced with salted butter along with your fruit, adding salt, starch, fat, and calories to your fruit to make a complete meal.

Better yet, do all those things.

What really matters is that you don't overdo the fluids, or at least that you become cognizant of how food interacts with your body to the extent that you can start mastering it and staying in a nice high metabolism, low stress "zone" all the time.

The biggest help is just making sure to salt food until it tastes "just right." Eat until you are full and satisfied of a variety of foods to ensure adequate calorie intake. Then drink or eat something juicy like fruit when you are thirsty but never beyond your physical thirst unless it's in anticipation of a hot day outdoors or a tough workout or something. That's really about all there is to it. I know it sounds simple but that's the point. The answers to better health, I have found, are mostly found in the simple realm. And there is no better guide to anything than our own tastes, appetites, and thirsts. Disobeying our bodies' cries for certain things, overriding our instincts, and exerting stubborn willpower is where we create the most damage, generally-speaking.

Anyway, I hope the inclusion of that section didn't do your head in with too many details. But I promise it is worth your while, especially if you are urinating frequently and have been for years due to the restrictive eating and stress you've been exposed to, to really pay attention to your food to fluid ratio. Get some yellow color back into that wee-wee, man. It should be yellow enough that, if you were to pee in the snow, people walking by it later would know not to eat it.

Even a single episode of frequent urination or just a strong, sudden urge to urinate out of nowhere, including having to get up and pee at night (which you shouldn't have to if things are really working right – and no it's probably not your bladder or your prostate regardless of what your doctor may have told you), is a strong cue to eat a dry, carbohydrate-rich, salty snack.

While it may seem silly if you've never paid much attention to these things, I ask you to do at least one thing – pay attention to how much colder your hands and feet are when your urine is clear vs. when it is yellow. It will be more noticeable to some than others, and a few rare cases may actually feel warmer with pale urine. But when you start to connect this dot, you'll really see why my work has taken me away from the small, trifling matters of nutrition and guided me to the bigger, more significant aspects of basic human physiology.

Anyway, don't drink too much, and don't eat too much watery food until your metabolism has come up. When it has you can, and should, drink far more fluids and return to eating more of the quintessential watery health foods – all those soups and salads and smoothies and crap, as long as you can do so without seeing body temp quickly retreat. For now, eat your calories and only drink as much as required to keep from getting dehydrated. What should you drink? Well, anything but plain water for at least the first few weeks. Make sure whatever you drink has some calories in it, and be flexible in your thinking. Many ill people have very high potassium to sodium ratios in their blood, and soft drinks and Gatorade treat them far better than fruits and juices and smoothies and coconut water and all that stuff your mind tells you is "healthier."

Exercise Rehab

S trap yourself in, as this chapter is going to go on forever. I love writing about exercise for starters (maybe because my metabolism is high), and have a lot to say about it. This chapter is not just a black and white do this and do that kind of party either. We'll delve into rehabilitating your relationship with exercise, as many people in the modern world are doing way too much or way too little. The ones doing a lot often are doing it for all the wrong reasons (to achieve or maintain starvation-level energy deprivation). And we will most certainly delve into the quantity or "dosage" and type of exercise that is best for someone recovering from a low metabolism. I'll share a few words about the role of exercise in health beyond the recovery period as well.

Exercise. Depending on who you are, the word alone is enough to evoke a wide spectrum of emotions. From a snooty disgust to a feeling of pride and accomplishment to a deep feeling of guilt – exercise is a massive topic on many levels.

As humans we are the only species that thinks about what we eat, and whether or not it is good for us. We are also the only species that can create intellectual interference regarding physical activity. On one hand, this interference is a good thing. We can use our minds to invent exercise strategies that allow us to become much more in terms of strength, endurance, athleticism – than we ever could be just by walking around looking for some food. But it of course has a dark side too, because, unlike a dog that is always eager to run and jump and play, we humans can convince ourselves that exercise is a bad, uncomfortable, and unpleasant thing. And almost never do it.

Dieting paired with exercise, and the defeatism that leads to when you fail at reaching some level of mythical hotness, tends to create a lot of negative vibes around exercise. When exercise is treated like a necessary evil to accomplish some other goal, and especially when it doesn't work as it so often doesn't, exercise gets thrown out as a tiresome, boring, ineffective way to spend one's time.

In such a scenario, it has basically become looked at as "work," or something you do against your will in order to obtain something else. A relationship between a person and exercise becomes more like the relationship between a garbage man and garbage. And I'm pretty sure there wouldn't be any more garbage men if they stopped getting paid to do it. If you have made exercise into work, and you're not seeing any payouts for it such as feeling good and looking like you want to look from it, why bother? It doesn't take a whole lot of mundane "calorie-burning" on a piece of cardio equipment before this type of relationship takes root.

Or maybe your aversion to exercise is deeper and more subtle than just failed attempts at losing weight and keeping it off. Perhaps you weren't a very good athlete growing up. Instead of accepting that you were a useless good-for-nothing, you probably found something else to become good at and take pride in yourself for. Maybe you got great grades and could play three instruments while all those "dumb jocks" were running around being unproductive. Choosing to look down upon exercise and exercisers could very well be a self-defense mechanism that you used to build up your own self-esteem long ago – only strengthened when seeing a bunch of people a lot more attractive than you coming in and out of the gym as an adult ("Oh, those narcissistic numbskulls – running on their hamster wheels instead of doing something to positively contribute to society!").

What would the alternative have been? To sit around moping about how ugly, weak, slow, and uncoordinated you naturally are? I don't think so. Having some self-esteem is important, and self-esteem basically comes down to feeling like you are gifted in ways that others aren't. Doing lots of exercise would have just given you more of a reminder of areas that you aren't the least bit gifted.

We won't go fully down that rabbit hole, but if you truly hate even the thought of exercise, those ideas hopefully will give you a few leads on why that might be. Explore them. Get to the bottom of your disordered relationship with moving your body around. When you get there, think of some of the ways you have been both benefited and harmed by having a distaste for exercise. When you start to feel more neutral about the idea of improving your own fitness, compared to no one else but yourself, and done for the sake of doing it rather than as a means to measure up to a level of leanness that may be out of reach for your body type and physical makeup, then you're about ready to actually do some of it. Hey, maybe there isn't any deep reason, you just really like video games and Facebook, and your desire to stay glued into those suppresses any natural desires you may have to move around.

I will say that I found a website the day before writing this that had all the old-school Nintendo video games on it. I got plenty of exercise. My vocal cords especially. They haven't had a workout like that in a long time. Ever tried to play Tecmo Super Bowl using the Seahawks? Yeah, it's frustrating. Dave Krieg can barely keep his passes in the field of play, much less hit a wide open Tommy Kane 75 yards downfield.

Having flirted with near-total glorification of exercise, as it seems pretty evident that the majority of our modern society does too little of it, it's time to point out that there is an even more debilitating side to exercise. Overdoing it. And, when combining overdoing it with underdoing your eating as is recommended by generally everyone in the weight loss and fitness industry, a lot of metabolic damage is done.

The original versions of this book called for a complete reprieve from any and all serious exercise (the heavy breathing kind you could call it) for at least a month. And taking an extended break from exercise is extremely therapeutic for some. I personally come from an absolutely insane overexercising past, involving weeks and even months at a time of very intense hiking and cycling up to 10 hours a day. For me, when I finally took a few months off just to feed myself well and relax as much as possible (living in Maui for that, which REALLY helped!), it was life-changing on much more than just a physical level. I had been playing drill sergeant inside my head to push myself to my physical limits for over a decade. It was a long overdue snoozefest on the beach.

But I don't think there's any need to take it to such an extreme, and exercise can probably improve most people's metabolic function when the type and dosage is right as we will discuss in just a sec. After all, quality exercise increases the number of mitochondria in the muscles, those little energy powerhouses that determine metabolic rate and the general youthfulness of one's bodily function.

Obviously each person's situation and history is unique, and how people take the advice to do some exercise is all very different on the individual level. I think the best thing to consider when making your own personal decision to start or continue exercising through your own metabolic recovery period is to assess how much of a role exercise excess played in your own demise, and how severely impaired your metabolism is. Recovering from a severe eating disorder or cease to have a menstrual period for the last couple of years? By all means, stop exercising completely. But for your average chronic dieter looking to do some smaller repair work, this simply isn't necessary. As with anything, there is a spectrum of severity, and only you can decide where you fall on that spectrum.

Now, onto the discussion of exercise itself...

Exercise means many things to many people, and I think exercise can be factored into a person's life very healthfully in a multitude of ways. Some will get a lot more exercise if they don't do any formal "workouts" at all. In fact, some research that I've come across over the years even suggests that people who don't "exercise" move around a lot more and are actually more physical than those who follow structured workouts. I believe it. When I'm doing very little working out I end up moving around a lot more, and finding things to do physically like play basketball or go on walks – when otherwise I might be too damn tired from my 30-minute workout to feel the inclination to do those things.

This is especially true when living in an interesting place during the good-weather months. If I were living in Colorado like I did for so many years, I would be out hiking, fishing, skiing, snowshoeing – doing all kinds of things outdoors purely for fun. I know hardly anyone that "works out" in the area I grew up in, and everyone living there looks great (I actually toyed with the idea of including a random Facebook photo of a friend of mine with her girlfriends as visual proof, but what little conscience I have spoke up and made me delete it). There is no obesity epidemic at all in the small mountain communities where I spent my late teenage years and most of my 20's. But if I were to go and purposely work out while living in such an interesting place with so many interesting physical things to do, my excitement for doing those things would probably be met with a sudden urge to visit YouTube followed by a nap.

However, I live in Florida now and there's only so many times you can walk up and down a pancake-flat beach before you get a little antsy to do something more challenging. Living in Florida, I have to have more structured exercise or I just won't do enough to keep from getting progressively less fit. I'm not a big swimmer, my past as an athlete has left me completely over the idea of participating in any competitive sports, and the cheap gyms near my home make it a no-brainer. The gym is the place for me and my current life situation.

So, the first thing when pursuing any type of exercise is to make it authentic to you. If you would rather express yourself physically through gardening, paddle surfing, and yoga, then by all means, carry on. If you like the gym and get a lot out of your time in there, that's great too. The most impressive bodies young and old are almost always found inside a gym, and those bodies are doing a lot less total exercise than the bodies that get their activity in through various forms of recreation.

But odds are, living in the peculiar modern world that we do, exercise is something that you probably find yourself sort of having to squeeze in efficiently. That doesn't have to be a bad thing though, as there are many advantages to our modern exercise world if you actually put all that fancy equipment to work for you.

I'd like now, if you'll indulge me, to talk about a few important aspects of exercise that you may not hear elsewhere. There's obviously a million perspectives and tips and snippets about exercise out there, but these are some of the things I've come to prioritize. Like magic diets, there are plenty of magic exercises and programs out there too – and if you don't prioritize and focus on a few important basics you'll drive yourself mad pinballing back and forth between exercise ideologies no different than your forays into diet ideologies…

Progress-oriented Exercise

Being physically fit and feeling strong are priceless attributes. Not only does most information out there validate that the net result of attaining and maintaining a good level of fitness and strength is fantastically healthy and beneficial to your overall quality of life as you age – metabolically and otherwise, but also there is something inherently exciting and inspiring about being in top form. These confident feelings are worth their weight in gold in terms of how they translate to the total life experience. We all want to be there. We are all inspired by feats of human strength and athleticism. I think it's a beautiful thing to take action and perform at your best by getting fit and strong. At the very least I know it wounds you on a deep level every time you have difficulty climbing a flight of stairs or standing up when you're not at your fittest.

When it comes to actually achieving it though, just going and pumping your arms around at a gym and logging some miles on a treadmill don't do much. Sure, maybe for a month or two you see some results, or reclaim results previously earned, but then things have a way of petering out. The exercise starts to feel increasingly pointless as you put in work, day after day, week after week, only to look and perform at the exact same level.

"Progress" is one of my favorite words. When we feel progress, life is good. When we don't, life feels flat. When you want to head in a certain direction with your life and then definitively start to take action and see yourself moving in that direction, the worries and fears really fade away.

Progress is very important when it comes to physical training, and I prefer to see people put all of their emphasis on it. Most people really want to look strong and fit, but because the changes when you are doing it without starving yourself have a tendency to be so slow and gradual as to be almost completely imperceptible – it's hard to stick with it for very long. If you don't see progress, and you don't feel it, the drive to continue is quickly extinguished.

That's why, when it comes to progress, it's really important to track progress in an almost scientific manner. That way you can actually SEE the improvement. You can also see when there is no improvement or even some regression, which is a valuable piece of information when it comes to designing and dosing your exercise, and also an important clue that you may be doing more harm than good with the type and quantity of exercise that you're doing.

Tracking progress carefully also allows you to move towards a stronger and fitter version of yourself at a much safer and more sustainable pace. You don't have to rush so that you are changing so fast you can see the difference from day to day. Rushing to fitness is a huge problem, and causes a really high burnout rate. Gyms know this, which is why they go ahead and sell many times as many gym memberships as they have room in their gym for members. Rather, you should strive for slow and steady improvements and be doing slightly LESS, not more exercise than you can tolerate. As I often say, "The best kind of exercise is the kind you'll still be doing ten years from now." And the biggest factor for sticking with something for that long is always having a good exercise appetite. Doing a little less than you're capable of keeps you ever-hungrier for more, and there's nothing to burn out from or wagon to fall off of.

Just as important as your exercise appetite is the fact that always staying fresh and fully recovered and eager to kick butt insures continual progress. Progress is rarely the result of dragging your tired and depleted body into the gym for a forced workout. Progress comes from pushing yourself to new heights, and that is something that comes from being fresh and fired up.

Yes of course you'll make more progress in the first 3 months if you do tons of work. But this is not a race to see who can get the fittest in 3 months. This is not that Body for Life thing or whatever that's called. Rather, your fitness pursuits are meant to be perpetually productive. And if you go too hard for a few months and then fizzle out, repeating that again and again, you'll get precisely nowhere. In my experience, intermittent overexercising spritzed with long periods of sedentary recovery (like 6 months) is a great way to get fat, lose some self-confidence in your ability to follow through on a goal, and dislike exercise more and more every year.

The way to actually get substantially stronger and fitter, with the extremely high probability that you will look substantially stronger and fitter to go along with that, is, quite simply, to stick with it. Stick with it yes, and of course make steady progress month after month for years. The key to sticking with it is to…

1. Not get hurt
2. Not overdo it
3. Do things that you like that are also convenient

4. Track progress to reassure that your efforts are paying off

And that's about it. Now let's talk about exercise specifically and how that ties into metabolism. Plus I just want to share with you a few exercise hacks that I've accumulated over the years to help you get more benefit from it with less time and effort.

In *Diet Recovery I*, I introduced a concept called MAXercise – a specific variety of high intensity interval training (HIIT). While in theory interval training is great – done with short bursts of maximum effort followed by recovery, followed by another round up to 10 total rounds – in actuality I find really high intensity stuff too difficult to consistently face. Going to the threshold of your abilities is extremely difficult to have courage for. I just can't do it. I don't expect you to either. There are some places of high intensity that just aren't realistic for all but the most barbarically self-loathing, which are the people that need that type of training the LEAST!

So, while the research will probably continue to show that the harder you push yourself in high-speed bursts of grueling intensity, research is really irrelevant to being a real, living, breathing human being. Of course, by now you've already gathered that I feel that way. But with exercise, research is just not as important as big words like "sustainable" and "realistic."

But, having said that, it does seem that most scientific research is congruent – short, hard workouts are better than long, easy ones. So if you are going to do something, whatever it is, you'll probably get better results from doing it vigorously. How vigorously? Well, depends on how healthy you are. The more solid your metabolism, the better your sleep and lower your stress, and the younger you are – generally the more intensely you can exercise without any ill effects. If you are in shambles and haven't exercised in ages, just start out nice and easy and slow and build intensity over time. A good rule of thumb starting out is to exercise at an intensity level where you can still breathe through your nose.

Let's talk more specifically though about this general concept. Because we all know what a treadmill is, we will use it as a baseline for discussion.

On a treadmill you could do a nice, easygoing workout for 30 minutes. In that 30 minutes the treadmill tells you that you burned 150 calories. How many calories you burn has no bearing on weight loss or anything like that, but the calories burned is the best total metric for how much work you performed. Or, you could do the same 30-minute workout on the treadmill but do it a lot more vigorously, burning 225 calories in the same period of time. This could be done at a steady pace, or you could be doing intervals wavering back and forth between really hard and easy enough to catch your breath. Regardless, you have just increased your intensity, and the workout will no doubt be more productive for increasing your fitness levels, which is really what matters in the grand scheme of things. Increased fitness is the goal.

X The most frequent mistake that people make, however, is keeping the intensity level the same but increasing the duration and increasing *endurance* not necessarily fitness, speed, power, or strength. This is a problem for many reasons. One is that your fitness doesn't necessarily improve just because you can go longer at the same low level of intensity. Secondly, making progress in the form of increased endurance leads to more and more and more training to infinity. That's not practical for many people, nor is it particularly kind on the body to be out doing something like jogging for 10 or more miles several times a week. Maybe you can get away with that, but I know I can't. And where do you go once you've run 15 miles? 20, then 25, then 30, then 35...?

From a metabolism standpoint, increasing endurance but not speed and power is even more backwards. Increasing endurance generally lowers basal energy production/metabolism. It brings about a set of adaptations that are really at odds with what most people want to achieve in terms of health, resting metabolism, and body composition. What slow, steady, long-duration exercise at a low to moderate intensity level does is encourage the body to become more efficient. While "efficient" is a word with a positive connotation, when it comes to our bodies, efficiency is more like an economy car, which, in order to save money on gas, has to sacrifice speed and power.

Speed and power is a totally different adaptation, and by the same token worsens endurance. Having strong, hard, powerful muscles and heavy, dense bones does not lend itself well to long-duration activity. You burn too many calories and do too much work to be good at endurance activities. To be good in endurance activities you must be able to travel efficiently. The best marathon runners and triathletes are the ones who, if I had to venture a guess, can burn fewer calories per mile, and thus not run into a depletion of energy reserves for hours. Burning fewer calories per mile is about having a low metabolic rate, low temperature, low muscle mass, low organ and bone weight, and so forth – being borderline emaciated basically.

Even more concerning, endurance exercise, and the adaptations the body undergoes in response to be better equipped for long duration activity, is totally in opposition to great hormonal health. In men, testosterone drops. In females, progesterone plummets. You also big rises in baseline cortisol, drops in DHEA, and other alarming trends. All of these changes come about to help break the body down into a lighter, weaker, poorly-performing machine designed to simply be able to do slow exercise with less caloric expenditure.

That's all a dramatic oversimplification of course, spritzed with exaggeration, but I want you to grasp such a concept and be open to the idea of training more for speed, power, and strength. I think you'll be glad you did, not only for the health benefits and the results you may visibly see and feel from doing it, but because it saves a hell of a lot of time and does a lot less wear and tear on your body – all while increasing, not decreasing, your fertility, sex drive, hormonal health, immune system strength, and more – assuming you aren't overdoing it.

Back to the treadmill talk. I've bashed treadmills and a lot of standard cardio equipment in the past. I think a lot of health and exercise gurus do this to sound cool and to establish themselves as being unique in a sea of mindless exercising sheep. In actuality, it's not the piece of equipment or type of exercise you're doing as much as it is the quality of the work you are putting into it. And a treadmill, just like any modern or primitive piece of exercise equipment barring perhaps the Thigh

Master, can be a great tool to achieve better fitness if you let it.

Earlier we talked about higher intensity levels on a treadmill, and how 225 calories burned in 30 minutes represents more intense exercise than 150 calories in 30 minutes. Great. So how would you go about increasing your fitness in a progress-oriented way on a treadmill or similar piece of equipment? Easy – keep the time the same, but try to get increasingly more work accomplished in that same amount of time. In this case burning more calories in the same half hour, or 20 minutes, or 10 minutes, or even just a few minutes. Progress is progress. If you can do more work in the same amount of time, you are moving in the right direction.

Over the period of say, 12 months, your calories burned in 30 minutes on a treadmill might look something like this. Each number represents calories burned in a 30-minute workout...

January – 170, 182, 189, 196, 203, 206
February – 210, 215, 219, 221
March – 227, 229, 230, 230, 238
April – 244, 245, 246, 255, 255
May – 255, 255, 260, 262
June – 264, 265, 267
July – 272, 280, 281, 283
August – 288, 294, 295
September – 290
October – 272, 279, 283, 288, 294
November – 296, 300, 303, 311, 313, 316
December – 319, 327, 331, 340

Notice above that training isn't necessarily robotic. In August and September you can see that workouts dropped, and progress dipped a little from taking some time off from exercise. Then, suddenly, progress picks back up at a much higher rate after taking some rest. This is all part of pursuing progress as well. Sometimes a one step back, two steps forward approach is in order. You will go through up and down cycles. You will also see that sometimes training less yields bigger leaps in performance, especially as you get faster and faster. What matters is that the trend is generally on its way up over time. And, sure enough, even though one workout was just slightly better than the last, work output in a 30-minute timespan increased from 170 to 340 in a year, a doubling of fitness by that yardstick – and done with 30-minutes an average of once per week or so.

This is just one example at how progress can be tracked. Even if you were to do this in just a 5-minute workout and work on increasing speed or work capacity in that 5-minutes, you could still track progress and get significantly fitter. What, you don't think you would be significantly fitter in the process of going from running a half mile in 5-minutes to a full mile in 5-minutes over a year or two of training? To be perfectly honest, doing even shorter workouts has some advantages, because the shorter the duration the higher you can ramp up the speed. The benefits of exercise do not come from burning calories. The benefits of exercise come from the hormonal adaptations the body makes to better handle the demands being placed upon it. And these adaptations come from doing very hard work – not very long work. The shorter the workout, the harder you can work. By definition, to increase the duration of an activity you must decrease the intensity, and when intensity goes down, results diminish – generally-speaking.

I hope you are getting the basic concept here. I want you to heal your metabolism AND get in great physical shape. I don't think the two goals are mutually exclusive.

There are infinite ways to do this too. Like I said, I just used a treadmill as an example because we all know what that is and it makes this all easier to conceptually grasp.

An even better way to get fit might be to set up a little bodyweight circuit – let's say 10 pushups, 10 bodyweight squats, 10 burpees, 3 pullups, and a plank hold for 30 seconds. You could do 5 rounds of this and time how long it takes you to get through the workout, trying to get the same amount of work done in increasingly less time to insure progress. Maybe the first time it takes you 30 minutes. Over a year you manage to get that down to just 15 minutes for 5 rounds through – you definitely got a lot fitter.

Or maybe you add more and more rounds of the circuit, and make progress that way – going from 5 rounds in 30 minutes to 10 rounds completed in 30 minutes over the course of a year. That works too.

Better yet, do a combination of things to keep it fresh, keep it challenging, and work your body in a variety of ways for greater mobility and athleticism. Whatever you choose is fine as long as you like it, don't do too much of it, don't get hurt, and make progress in the manner described.

Strength Training

Let's now turn to strength training, as this is a vital part of fitness, and is probably the best form of structured exercise one can do from a metabolism point of view. With some special hacks that I have for you on strength training, you'll really get a lot out of it, dramatically increase your strength in the basic lifts in just a few months, be doing some strength training at most once every two weeks at the end of the first year (and still progressing), and never get so much as winded doing it (unless you just want to).

For how to achieve this, let's go back to a statement made several paragraphs back: *"By definition, to increase the duration of an activity you must decrease the intensity, and when intensity goes down, results diminish – generally-speaking."* Nowhere is this more apparent than with strength training. You can lift little featherweight girly pink dumbbells all over the sky, and it won't make but a tiny bit of difference in your strength levels – if you notice any improvement at all. The reason is because the muscle's strength isn't being challenged. To increase your strength, the key is to put your strength to the test. Then rest until fully recovered (3-30 days depending on how strong you are) and do it again.

Interestingly, the more sets you do, and the longer the duration of the sets (thus requiring a lighter weight), the less strength gains you will get – because longer duration and lighter weight = less intensity and less stimulus for strength development. This may not be true for everyone, and the things we will discuss may not be the ultimate form of all training, but it's enough to get large results with small effort. It's things like this in life that get my attention. Hell, I can't even unload the dishwasher. And I know you, with a much busier life than mine, will probably be even more overjoyed to have been exposed to the following information.

What all that means is that the heavier the weight you use, the shorter the set. The shorter the set, generally the easier it feels. I mean, how exhausted can you get in 5 seconds, really? You can't even get out of breath doing it. And, working with great precision in your training, there's really not much of a need to do multiple sets.

Maybe you're not getting what I'm saying here. What I'm saying is that if you want to see the most rapid progress in strength gains, do one 5-second set of a handful of basic exercises once every 3-30 days depending on how strong you are. The stronger you are, the more damage you do and the more time it takes for you to effectively recover – recovery defined here as being stronger than you were last time you performed the exercise.

No, I'm serious. I haven't lost my mind. Now let's describe what this 5-second set looks like. It takes about 5 seconds or so to do one repetition with the maximum weight you are capable of lifting. Only problem here is that lifting as much weight as you possibly can through a full range of motion repetition is extremely dangerous, which violates Stick With It rule #1 – Don't get hurt. Well, that's not the only problem. The other problem is that if you do a full-range repetition in say, bench press, with 200 pounds – that 200 pounds is only hard to press for the first few inches off of your chest. The rest of the repetition is much easier because you have better and better leverage the straighter your elbows get. With my elbows straight I can bench press about 425 pounds, so 200 isn't exactly a maximum weight at that portion of the rep. To do a 1-rep max through the full range of motion I have to drop the weight to 230 or so, almost half the weight of what I can press in the strongest portion of the exercise.

Anyway, I won't bore you with all the minutiae there. This is not an exercise book. Suffice it to say that there is a way around the danger of working with heavy loads, and a way to truly test your absolute max strength each time you go to work out – do static holds.

Static holds

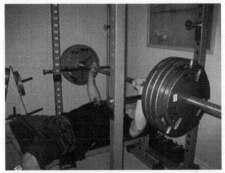

Instead of actually doing a "normal" repetition of an exercise, with a static hold you load up as much weight as you can while still being able to lift and hold a heavy weight in place. I don't think it matters too much at what point in your range of motion that you are doing the static hold, as long as it is the maximum weight you can hold for roughly 5 seconds. If you can hold it for more than 10 seconds, you didn't use enough weight and should add some until you can only hold it for just about 5 seconds. You record the weight used, and then go in and try to do more weight the next workout in each of the exercises you select to do this with.

Here is a picture of what it looks like to do a static hold for bench press. Simply lift the weight off of the rack, hold it as long as you absolutely can with all the might you can muster, and then set it back down. Done.

Great exercises to do would be some kind of leg exercise – squat or leg press, dead lift, shoulder press, lat pulldown, bicep curls, shrug, and calf raises for a total of about 8 exercises – one hold for 5 seconds each. Of course you can do a little accessory work too – like a set of hard abs work and a couple other odds and ends.

That's all there is to it. Just make sure that you use something like a Power Rack (shown in image) or Smith machine (similar) for exercises like the bench press to make sure you don't crush yourself with the weights you are using. Record the weights used and make sure you are getting stronger with EVERY workout.

The key to getting stronger with every workout, making consistent progress for many months and even years on end, is to properly space your workouts. When you are starting out and pretty weak, you can do a workout like this as often as once every four days and still get stronger every time. Then, after several workouts, you'll stop getting stronger and have to space it to once every five days. The stronger you get, the more recovery time you need because greater strength equals greater demands on the body equals more time to full recovery. Get strong enough and you might literally find that you need to keep your workouts to once a month to keep making progress.

If you have damaged your metabolism somehow, or you are just weakly constituted naturally, this really is the ultimate form of exercise. You make great progress with a minimum amount of strain. Your nervous system does not get worn down with such a small load of exercise. This approach to exercising is what proponents of high-intensity exercise call "the minimum effective dose" of exercise. If it takes a 5-second hold once every week or few to get stronger, and doing the typical 3 sets of 10 repetitions 3 times per week is less effective, why do more? For a really healthy person it's tough to justify the extra struggle and strain to lift weights several hours per week. For someone in recovery from having done some serious damage to themselves via dietary restriction and other stressors, doing more exercise volume is even more silly.

Although the book is filled with almost comical logic or lack thereof, the book *Train Smart* by Pete Sisco talks about this type of training in much greater depth than I can justify discussing in a book about improving your metabolism and getting off of the diet rollercoaster. Twisted logic aside, the training works for many, and is the best fit for someone trying to get the greatest reward from exercise with the least amount of self-punishment.

If this type of training, and the equipment used are unavailable to you, a similar substitute is to do the workout described in the book *Body By Science* by Doug McGuff and John Little (who is a close friend of Pete Sisco's). In BBS, you do one set of slow repetitions ranging from 60-90 seconds, for 3-5 exercises. Done. Add weight each workout and repeat on an increasingly-infrequent basis as described earlier.

If you have no access to a gym at all, and want to apply some of these same principles working out at home with minimal equipment, a decent substitute is to follow the home workouts in the book *Slow Burn* by Fred Hahn.

But any old strength training will do, and some strength training is better than no strength training at all. While many women may not identify with the idea of getting strong and lifting heavy objects, I highly recommend getting hypnosis or something like a slap across the face with a wet noodle to clear that erroneous bias out of your head. Strength training is the ultimate physique enhancer for both men and women (modern beauty standards are rapidly changing to even favor women with much more lean body mass and higher body mass index), and yields major health improvements for just about everyone – especially older people already showing signs of sarcopenia (muscle wasting) and osteopenia (bone loss). Thoughtful graphic that someone put together below…

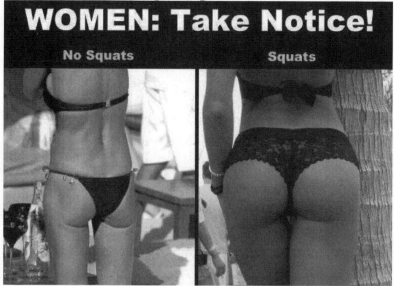

That pretty much concludes what I wanted to share with you about exercise. If you can just prioritize fitness and track progress, and strength and track progress – seeking out the minimum effective dose to keep improving with each, AND STICK WITH IT, I have no doubt you'll really get somewhere.

In addition to this structured training, play and have fun. Let all your other "exercise" be purely recreational and not something you do for any other purpose. With greater strength and fitness, you won't be able to keep yourself from moving around and doing things. Physical activity only sucks when you are out of shape or doing it as a form of work and not play.

Just make sure that you are exercising for the right reasons, not the wrong ones. The idea here is to obtain the health and metabolic benefits delivered by strength and fitness. The idea is to give your body a stimulus that it can adapt to for higher power, strength, and performance. The idea is to focus on improvements in the training itself and not look for it to have some immediate impact on your waist measurement. It probably won't. But if you stick with it long enough to really substantially improve, it almost certainly will. A change in body fat levels or not, you'll look and feel better and be more confident and healthy. Get past your inhibitions or your obsessive and self-detrimental exercise abuse – whatever haunts you, and get on track to doing it right in a way that is safe and sustainable.

At least try it. If you don't you'll think I'm totally nuts. If you do you'll be pretty shocked to see that the simple things I mentioned above work as well as or better than just about all the stuff you've tried in the past.

Or just convince yourself I'm crazy. Many people have done that over the years. Either way you'll eventually come around – not just with this exercise stuff but all of it. Because I'm right. And eating whatever the hell you want and doing minimalist training is way more funner than the (un)popular alternatives.

As a last word on exercise, and I really mean it this time I promise – let the biofeedback that we discussed earlier determine how much and what kind of exercise you should really be doing. I can't say in a book whether YOU should be doing a little or a lot, or even none. It's up to you to figure that out. If you start to experience strange aches and pains, sleep loss, frequent urination, cold hands and feet, a plummeting body temperature – well, you should know what that means. Something needs to change.

What to Expect

Excerpt from *Diet Recovery* on some topics we are about to discuss…

"As you start out, remember that you are challenging your metabolism, your glucose metabolism, your digestion, and more. This does not feel good!!! Headaches, skin breakouts, brain fog, severe drowsiness after meals, out-of-control hunger – particularly if you are coming off of a low-carb diet, heartburn and other digestive glitches – these are all normal in the first week or two. But just when you think you are poisoning yourself with all this food something pretty cool happens. You start to notice improvements in how your body handles everything. Instead of running from all these problem foods and big, heavy meals you experience your body rising to the challenge, making use of the tools you've given it, and functioning much, much better.
So be prepared to be challenged and have to muster up some resilience and persistence. This is not all fun and games. It's like trying to get back in shape after years of couch surfing. You get tired. You get sore. You ache. But it makes you stronger. You'll see."

I can't tell you exactly what will happen to you as you follow some of these general guidelines. I can't give you timelines on anything either. It all depends. It depends upon your age, your gender, your history, your genetics/constitution, and a lot more that just can't realistically be broken down for each individual. But there are some general things that happen to a large percentage of people when going through this process. I will speak in high percentages, meaning that what I say will happen for most. The peculiar stuff that most people don't seem to experience, I won't delve into. Here goes, starting with the uglier side of things…

Digestive Problems

At first, especially if your diet has been very limited for a long period of time, you will probably collide with some noticeable digestive disturbances. Even switching your dog from one brand of dog food to another is enough to cause digestive upsets for a few days before the digestive tract starts to acclimate to even this simple change. The change you are undergoing may be a heck of a lot more dramatic than switching from Purina to Ol' Roy. So don't let some bowel issues, bloating, acid reflux/indigestion, and other things throw you off course. Expect them, and gear up to be resilient when challenged by them. Remember, the objective isn't to find the safe foods that keep you from having digestive problems. Take that route and you'll eventually whittle your diet down to practically nothing. Rather, the objective is to improve your digestive abilities, and allow your digestive tract to adjust to eating pretty much anything and everything. This transition does take time. There are even digestive bacteria and enzyme systems that must do a Chinese Fire Drill of sorts for things to start running smoothly. But once this transition is made and your metabolism is ablaze, you should be digesting impossible combinations and quantities of food like a boss. This can take anywhere from a few days to more than a month.

Corpse-like Fatigue

When you go from being in a highly-stressed, underfed state to a de-stressed, overfed state, the adrenal glands pretty much go on vacation. You know how you feel after a big Thanksgiving feast? Your eyelids feel like they weigh a thousand pounds. You feel warm and cozy and tingly all over. All you want to do is pass out into a coma-like slumber. There's a good chance that you will spend a lot of time in this semi-comatose state for many weeks. Maybe even a whole month. If you are recovering from something really severe – like a major eating disorder, this phase can last much longer. Like a whole frickin' year. Don't beat yourself up for feeling utterly unproductive or freak out and think there's something wrong because you're not your former upbeat, energetic self. Spend some time in this state and welcome it openly. It's a healing place to be.

Endocrinologist and author Diana Schwarzbein had a big impact on me with this concept. She states that running on adrenaline and wearing yourself out actually feels really good – whereas rebuilding feels kinda lousy. Like your body and brain have all slowed down by half.

Glucocorticoids, our hormones of stress, can actually create euphoria in large quantities, and shutting them down can cause feelings of near-withdrawal. I have likened eating disorders to a drug dependency, in that eating, once you go beyond a certain point of starvation, actually takes away your internal stimulant meds and makes you feel totally crappy and depressed, with a foggy unfocused brain. Get ready for such feelings, and don't let them fool you into thinking that what you are doing is a disaster, like this woman that wrote to me who displayed all the NORMAL reactions to starting out on this program from a highly-dieted, low metabolic state…

"Eating per your suggestion has been the absolute worst thing I've ever done to my body ever. 3 years ago I lost 100 lbs exercising and eating healthy.

When I looked into your literature to see about the stress in my life, things took a massive nose-dive. I have gained over 12 lbs in 10 days, I feel sluggish and lethargic all the time, and I'm pissed as hell that my stress level has not gone down, and I continue to gain even though I've modified my diet to include more whole foods. I'm bloated, gassy, fatigued, sick, frustrated, and wish I'd never EVER done the "Salt, Sugar, Saturated Fat, Starch" diet you so eloquently sell in your trash literature.

This is nothing but exploitation of people who are sincerely trying to balance their lives. Thanks for the extra weight, Mr. Stone. Glad it worked for you, too bad it ▬▬ up the rest of us."

messes

Menstrual Mayhem

A woman's menstrual cycle is a very sensitive thing. While almost all women notice having more regular rhythms and an absence of all menstrual problems like PMS, water retention, cramping, and so forth – and nearly all women who have lost their periods see it return quickly, very peculiar things can happen to the menstrual cycle for the first few cycles. Chaos is a good word to describe it. It seems that changing the metabolism around represents some big core alterations, and it is not uncommon to have two periods in a month, have an exceptionally heavy or light period or two, pass heinous clots, and have nothing shy of true menstrual mayhem for the first, oh I would say 2-4 cycles after commencing <u>rest</u> and <u>refeeding</u>. As long as you're seeing improvements in many of the other metabolic indicators, don't be thrown off course by this or start seeking out remedies and other diets to "fix" these problems.

Acne/Breakouts

I could design four or five wonderful programs that would make your skin as clear as an anorexic's urine. Zero carb, juice fasts, no-sugar diets – there are plenty. The problem is that most of those approaches, if you are to return to eating everything mixed together like a normal person, will make the skin worse than ever before. If other people can eat everything in sight without having big acne explosions, so can you. It's just a matter of getting your body to function properly.

Well, that's pretty much the pep-talk I give for those worried about re-developing acne when doing the rest and refeeding thing. Some are pleasantly surprised that their acne does not return at all, others do see acne quite aggravated at the start.

If you do notice some breakouts on your face and/or body, expect this to worsen for 1-4 weeks before it stabilizes. Then the skin should become progressively less inflamed until the acne problem clears up and maybe even gets better than it has been in years, with smooth and soft skin. Do not give up on being able to eat all macronutrients and all types of foods with good skin. It is possible to overcome even lifelong tendencies in any area, especially the skin.

Aches and Pains

When refeeding there is often some initial water retention, which can increase physical pain, as well as some pain related to other mechanisms. One of our primary anti-inflammatory internal pain medicines is cortisol. As I mentioned earlier, the adrenal glands that manufacture this cortisol more or less go on vacation. Sometimes there is a transient and temporary period of up to a month or two where pain levels are somewhat higher – especially in joints with a history of aching. Sometimes a small amount of aspirin can work as a reasonably safe pain-reliever.

Changes in Body Composition

When your temperature is below normal, consider yourself primed for some fat gain. From the time temperature is low until the time it reaches the ideal, you are much more likely to gain fat. But it's not all so simple and cut and dry as to think that you will just blimp up doing this. There's a lot more going on underneath the surface.

Before we go any further, it's very important to know, definitively, that our bodies possess an elaborate energy-regulating system. Attempts to consciously override that system usually result in a great deal of backlash, one form being of course a reduced metabolic rate. Another is a reduction in hormones of youth (progesterone, testosterone, DHEA, thyroid, etc.) that have a known tendency to steer ingested food towards the production of muscle tissue, bone, blood, heat, and energy – and an increase in the hormones that favorably steer ingested food towards fat cells (like cortisol).

All the hormones just mentioned are primarily controlled by command central for energy regulation, which is the hypothalamus in the brain. It's not like these hormones act in isolation. But command central doesn't just spin a giant wheel of metabolic fortune to determine how energy should be regulated at random. There are many different factors, a lot of them set into motion before we are even born, such as the number and size of fat cells. The biggest messenger of information regarding energy status comes from hormones like leptin that actually reside in our fat tissue. Pretty novel design actually, as falling body fat levels send a scarcity signal, and rising body fat levels send an abundance signal.

Of course, for reasons not entirely understood by modern science, many a person's hypothalamus is not getting this signal. Regardless of weight or past tendencies or scientific mysteries surrounding "leptin resistance" or any of that, I've found everyone universally responding in the same way to intentional and strategic dietary surplus – the abundance signal is sent. Metabolism rises substantially. Rate of weight gain descends until it stops altogether – usually coinciding with the body temperature reaching "normal."

X So, you will probably gain some weight at first, and most of it will be fat and water (the tendency to have edema, or water retention, is much greater the lower the metabolic rate). The weight gained that matters is the fat itself, as hormones in the fat tissue are what send this abundance signal to the brain, in turn

132

rearranging your hormonal landscape to one much more conducive to health and good functioning in all the main body systems (digestive, reproductive, cardiovascular, osmoregulatory, and so on). So don't try to necessarily avoid fat gain. That's like trying to become wealthy by avoiding money. Fat is where it's at.

X This fat initially accumulates at a much faster rate around the abdomen than other areas of the body during metabolic recovery. Some think this is due to the body's desire to add fat around the internal organs to protect them from hypothermia (low body temperature). In the past I figured it was to provide an energy supply to the internal organs. It doesn't really matter why. What matters is that it's going to happen during the first part of your diet recovery, and that you need to be prepared for it – not freaking out and getting nervous and jumping ship before the next wave of changes.

So, at the start you'll gain weight quickly, then it will slow, and then it will stop altogether. You might only gain weight for two weeks. You might gain weight for several months – maybe 15 pounds the first month, 10 pounds the second, 5 pounds in the third, and then finally none by the fourth month. I recommend just getting the weight gaining part over with. Gaining fat is horrifying. When you stop gaining weight, it's quite a relief and you can focus more on completing your recovery. I call the point of reaching zero fat gain eating enormous quantities of even the most palatable and "fattening" food as becoming "fat-proof." Fat-proofing yourself is a very important first step.

X It's also really important to take this process to completion. At first you gain weight around the abdomen, but then you fill out in the rest of your body – adding more subcutaneous fat, which is generally believed to be highly protective and actually healthy. Meanwhile, more and more of your weight gain consists of restored organ mass, bone mass, muscle mass, and glycogen storage. In other words, the LAST 10 pounds you may gain during recovery are the most important pounds. Those pounds restore you to full capacity and also improve how your body looks aesthetically.

Once all of that has taken place, and much of your abdominal fat has been redistributed throughout your entire body, and all your healthy tissue has been restored… THEN, you MAY start losing some body fat. Some do, some don't. But we as humans certainly have the mechanisms that enable the body to shed huge amounts of fat without any conscious effort to cut calories or burn more through exercise. Women after giving birth are a prime example, as they, without any conscious effort, often feel extremely hot and hypermetabolic while shedding 30-40 or even more pounds within the first six months of giving birth. Other women hold onto the weight but lose quite a bit once they stop lactating. It's just a matter of figuring out how to tap into your body's innate ability to do this effortlessly.

I can't, in good conscience, recommend you do anything other than continue to follow the high metabolism and good physical functioning where it leads, and see it through to the end of the cycle – even if it takes several years. I have a feeling, based on my own experience and that of others like personal trainer Billy Craig who has guided dozens of people through the process of high-calorie weight loss, that persistently maintaining a high metabolic rate and eating abundantly on a regular schedule while doing progress-oriented exercise, getting good sleep, and avoiding the yo-yo rollercoaster like the plague, that body fat will eventually come off.

If it does, great. If it doesn't, at least you're healthy and have made a very positive investment in your long-term well-being. One thing is for certain though, no diet or outrageous and unsustainable exercise regimen is going to fix the problem. What that will do is catapult your metabolism right back where it started and re-prime you for more fat gain above and beyond what you would have experienced had you just followed this process to completion. Resist the temptation to diet, and don't get wrapped up in quick weight loss. It will likely come back if you do anything to consciously force it off. In obesity research they refer to that as "intentional weight loss" and it has some nasty after-effects, including contributing to future weight gain past your starting point.

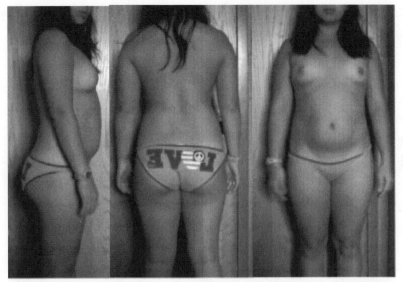

10-5-11 10am   135 pounds at 5'2"

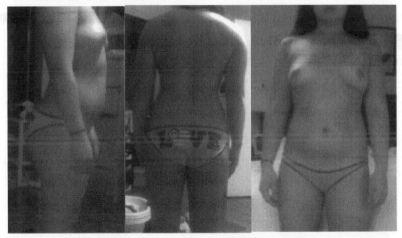

1-11-13 10am   143 pounds at 5'2"

Don't be too nervous though, or let me make you feel like the chances of success are too bleak and that you are forever going to have the body of Mr. Potatohead. They aren't really, and I think you'll find, as many do, that you eventually end up looking more muscular with more prominent fertile characteristics (a more masculine, muscular look for men – a more feminine hourglass figure and shapely look for women, with larger breasts and buttocks).

I don't have a lot of photo documentation for this, as I try to take the emphasis off of aesthetics – an obsession with them of course leading to this counterproductive dieting black hole in the first place, but I have included one example of a woman who, with a net gain of 8 pounds (I believe her weight peaked above 160 if I'm not mistaken) after completing this process, has seen remarkable improvements in the basic biomarkers of metabolism, and has also had her stomach flatten, her breasts become larger, and has much more of that hourglass figure – for her this whole process took about a year (the before photo is after doing lots of dieting and jogging). ▬▬▬▬ ▬▬
▬▬▬▬▬
(▬▬▬▬

Those are some of the more negative or frightening changes you will initially face when going through this. Now let's talk about some of the aspects of the recovery process that will be very welcomed and wonderful. We've mentioned some of these positive aspects of a high metabolism earlier, so we'll glide through them like a hard, high-metabolism penis through a gushing, slippery high-metabolism vagina (C'mon, after that picture how could I not be thinking in such metaphors, especially when she used the word "buckets" to describe the changes she's seen in vaginal lubrication in an email to me)…

Body Temperature Increase

Obviously you should experience an actual, genuine, increase in your body temperature. That was the objective when thatching this program together, fine-tuning it further and further over the years. How long will it take? Some see a big rise within the first 48 hours. Others see a slow, steady increase that takes place over many weeks and sometimes takes even a few months before temps get over 98F. Really going for it and eating recreationally of decadent foods, not feeling guilty about it or hesitant, hitting high calorie levels, getting great sleep, and being very consistent with it will dramatically accelerate the process. Not everyone is comfortable departing from dietary fears and ingrained patterns easily though, and that can really prolong the process.

Strength Increase

Whether you want to or not, you will gain muscle during this process (unless you are a bodybuilder taking time off), and you will gain strength. The primary purpose of this program is to put the body in a low-stress anabolic or growth state for an extended period of time.

Do some strength training as discussed, and you will likely gain strength twice as fast as you would under totally normal circumstances, and four or five times as fast as compared to not doing any training at all. When I went through a phase of very aggressive refeeding for three months I saw enormous increases in muscle size and strength beyond anything I have ever experienced – and I grew up with a weight room right next to my bedroom and was a competitive, hard-training athlete all the way to the collegiate level (meaning that I have done plenty of strength training in the past with minimal results – in the context of surplus calories and 10 hours of nightly sleep it actually worked!).

Harder, Stronger Teeth

Eat all the white sugar you want, but if you enter into a high-metabolic, low-stress state you are still going to see improvements in the strength and whiteness of your teeth – white sugar and all. Teeth have many similar characteristics to bone as to what influences their strength and overall health. When the body is in an anabolic, growth state you lay down fresh new minerals and protein in hard tissues like bones and teeth, and you should expect both to become significantly stronger. A couple people have even had fillings pop out and fresh new tooth fill into old cavities – something generally believed to be impossible.

At the very least you should notice a decrease in the sensitivity of the teeth. At first, eating sugar or drinking cold or hot drinks may cause a slight toothache. Continue and you probably will, as so many others have, start to notice that triggers of toothaches no longer give you any grief. I have a strange obsession with teeth and dental health, as I view this as being a great outwardly sign of health. I have always been very keen on how various physiological changes and diets impact the teeth – to the extent that I only brush my teeth once or twice a week to make sure nothing is off internally (because it manifests with tooth pain if there is).

There is an enormous amount of research both past and present showing the significance of healthy, strong, cavity-free teeth in overall health and degenerative disease resistance. Consider improvements here a huge positive investment in your overall well-being.

Increased Sex Drive and Function

I will refrain from going TOO much into detail after already crossing way beyond the border of appropriateness earlier, but increased appetite for sex and improvements in sexual function (better erections for men, as well as big increases in ejaculate volume and sperm motility... and more copious lube and increased fertility for women) are to be expected from a rise in metabolic rate. Noticing improvements in this department is a sure sign of moving in the right direction.

Softer, Moister Skin

With a rise in metabolic rate, especially if you take the advice not to drink excess fluids seriously, you will likely see an improvement in the softness and moisture of the skin. This is particularly true for those of you with the telltale low metabolism dry hands and lower legs/feet.

Calmer, More Stable Moods

Being well-fed is very conducive to feeling good-spirited, just as being hungry is a frequent trigger of irritability and dramatic mood swings – to the extent a new word was recently forged: "hangry." Your system generally should become more stable after an initial rollercoaster as you acclimate to the changes as well, keeping mood, energy levels, blood sugar levels, and body chemistry in general a lot more stable.

This brings up an important point that I haven't really squeezed in anywhere else – blood sugar stability is greatly tied to metabolic rate, as metabolic rate influences stored carbohydrate levels in the liver, general liver functionality, fatty acid levels in the blood, insulin sensitivity, glucocorticoids, and other known factors to heavily influence glucose metabolism. You don't have to live with "hypoglycemia" or what you perceive as blood sugar swings. You can overcome them, and feel completely stable and calm after giant double-portions of chocolate cake or whatever former hypoglycemic-trigger you wish to pillage. Even Broda Barnes went as far as to write a book on raising metabolic rate to overcome hypoglycemia in *Hope for Hypoglycemia*, and used cake as an example.

Better Sleep

When metabolism declines with age, sleep quality suffers. I believe that this is probably tied to the tug of war between metabolism and stress. Stress hormones like aldosterone and adrenaline peak at night, with peaks in cortisol in the early morning. The lower the metabolic rate, the more prominent these hormone surges become. One of the most common things to happen when metabolism is impaired is the onset of 2-4am wakeups and a need to urinate (stress hormones are diuretic in nature – making you pee) coinciding with the nightly peak in adrenaline. As metabolism gets increasingly lower, more frequent wakeups with more noticeable adrenaline side-effects are noted, such as erratic heart rhythms, anxiety attacks, excessive mental energy, serious nocturia (nighttime urination) and an inability to fall back asleep without food.

Average night sleep decreases with age, ranging from well over half the day in infancy to barely more than a third that much in senescence. Metabolism has a lot to do with the quantity and depth of sleep and this overall decline seen throughout the lifespan. When it rises, it is typical to experience greater sleep depth and quantity, and you should notice better sleep and feeling better rested too – sometimes instantly with a single day of hearty eating.

Improved Allergies and Food Sensitivities

Because semi-starvation and the resulting decline in metabolism causes intestinal permeability and increases the inflammatory response, amongst other undesirable changes…

"There is reason to believe that the epithelial lining of the gastrointestinal tract becomes more permeable to microorganisms in severe undernutrition. The morphological changes in the intestinal tract would strongly suggest this."
~Ancel Keys; *The Biology of Human Starvation*

…food allergies and intolerances are the norm, not the exception. While removing a problem food can be helpful in the short-term, if you take no action to stop the core reason why you are developing various hypersensitivities, expect to develop new ones, restrict some more, develop more, restrict some more – repeating until you have backed yourself in a corner and can hardly eat a thing.

I recommend, for most people, to look at dietary restriction as a last resort – not a first line of defense. Pulling certain foods (especially grains and dairy, which are the most socially and emotionally crippling because they are so prevalent in global diets, and they combine to make the best-tasting foods in existence) out of your diet is debilitating physically, psychologically, emotionally, and socially. You have my blessing to throw caution to the wind and eat everything, without restriction, and use the general attitude condoned here to improve your tolerance to certain things instead of resort to avoidance strategies.

Not everyone can overcome their dietary demons, but many are surprised to find that their food allergies and sensitivities were a result of a core dysfunction within their own bodies, and not something wrong with the food itself. This is truly a common result of rest and refeeding. If you can't eat a few foods, that's fine. You won't die from a gluten deficiency. But at least give it a try for the potential dietary freedom you could gain from an honest attempt to fix your natural hypersensitivity.

Loss of Cravings and Appetite Changes

For a typical person pursuing rest and refeeding, appetite initially goes berserk. You can't get enough food. Then appetite starts to mellow out a bit, and then food becomes downright disinteresting. That's all normal. I would follow your natural appetite cues through this process for the most part, unless, with a decline in appetite, you are seeing low metabolism symptoms come back with a vengeance and temperatures fall significantly. If that happens, it's probably best to eat whether you are hungry or not.

Cravings disappear much more quickly. Of course, if you are allowing yourself to eat foods that you've been restricting for a while, expect a pornographic sensation from eating them at first and an insatiable appetite for the forbidden food for a week or two. That's all normal. But cravings rarely persist beyond a week or two unless:

1. You are feeling guilty and remorseful about the food you crave and are now allowing yourself to eat
2. You are still restricting them in some way

If you have a long history with strong cravings for a certain food – like chocolate for example, or potato chips – you should overstock your house, car, desk at work… everything you can think of with this food until your state of arousal over it becomes neutralized. There's no reason to be haunted by any food. Lifelong cravings are a week away from permanently curing. Refeeding with all the foods one could desire or crave in ample abundance on a consistent basis eliminates this tendency, as well as the tendency to overeat or binge, without fail.

This physiological and psychological shift can go much deeper than just food cravings, but permeate into all addictions and compulsive behavior. When you experience this with food, and feel much greater inner stability, think about tackling some other vices while you're at it. Nobody likes to be enslaved to anything.

Well, except you sweet computer. We loves you Precious. Please don't destroy this book. We've worksis on it really hard (between games at www.nesforever.com, and amongst the 40 or so times we hitsis refresh per day on Google Analytics). We'll do anything you asksis of us.

Sorry that was lame. My brain is fried from all the YouTube videos I watched today. No I'm not addicted, I just don't leave the house most days or eat or do the dishes for weeks at a time because of all the youtube videos I need to catch up on. Plus, gotta hit that refresh button everywhere I can. Kinda cuts into my physical needs and social life. But like, seeing and talking to people in real life is so old school anyway. Hello! It's 2013! Get a Facebook account lmfao.

Redirecting Perfectionism

Well folks, I suppose it's about time to wrap this up. But you would be kidding yourself if you thought you were going to get away with reading a book about recovering from diets without taking a deeper look into the psychological makeup that got you in this mess in the first place. Oh yes, we're going there. We must. This is a piece that must not be left out.

One common trait found amongst those with eating disorders is perfectionism. It runs rampant in those that manage to beat down their body's inner drives with stubborn willpower to the point of actually endangering themselves. While I'm not suggesting that all dieters should start to believe they have eating disorders, I do believe that one very human desire catapults us into this in the first place...

The desire to be better.

Better than others. Better than ourselves in our current state.

Was that not what drove you to either pursue immortality or a more shapely figure through some type of metabolism-wrecking diet? I know that's how I got on this track. At 8 or 9 years old I began reading the labels on my breakfast cereal boxes, noting that there was a long list of vitamins, minerals, and fiber on their spines and numbers associated with each one. I began selecting only cereals with the highest percentages on them, and felt gratification and self-confidence over this "wise" choice. It was a chance to excel.

Later, amidst a sports-centric culture, I took a similar attitude towards exercise and began an even more powerful and self-destructive set of habits.

This ever-escalating trend of perfect eating and superhuman physical feats led me to the point of near-starvation out in the Wilderness, freezing cold, asexual, constipated, sleepless, incessantly urinating, beyond hungry, emotionally unstable, and alone, much like Chris McCandless – the subject of Jon Krakauer's book *Into the Wild*.

The only other thing I can think of as a substantial driver of dieting would be fear – I certainly encounter a lot of people who see someone die of a nasty disease and want to take better care of themselves, at least in part out of straight fear. Of course, with their desire to be healthier, they are misled by the popular, eating-disordered purveyors of nutrition advice and their delusions of grandeur – and steered down a dark tunnel to metabolic oblivion. This is followed by illness, and an intensified desire to eat and live perfectly.

Either way, a desire to be perfect, or at least better, is the spark that takes even the simplest desire to have better health and eventually turns it into a runaway freight train plowing straight over the lives we had once hoped to improve.

This first major thing I want to share with you in this arena is that you must let the idea of perfection as it pertains to your physical body go. If you can't let go of that, you will always fail in some way or another, even when you succeed.

The basic 'program' for lack of a better word almost invariably helps people to function better in some if not all of the most important physical competencies (digestion, sex, mood, sleep, strength, metabolism, dental health, etc.). But no one ever functions perfectly. Or looks perfect. Or lives forever. Or fails to see a decline with advancing age.

Use this program to restore some basic functionality – to the point where you can feel good enough to do the things you want to do in life. Then do them. Leave this dieting shit behind for good. Even forget about your physical appearance for the most part. The more headspace you can take away from such things, the healthier and better-looking you will likely become as you stop doing the very dieting that is counterproductive beyond compare.

As I've said many times and in many places, "You have to solve your weight problem to lose weight, not lose weight to solve your weight problem." In other words, stop thinking about losing weight and dieting and various ways to force the weight off – and having the very thoughts that there is something wrong with you, and you might actually see some real improvements when you least expect them.

Yes, it's easy to get momentarily fired up and believe that you really can, indeed, transcend the negative emotions tied to your body image. Actually doing it consistently is another thing entirely. I have a few words to share on this, and then we will move on to the most important thing I have to get across in this chapter – which is finding a replacement to fill the time and energy in your life.

As far as looks are concerned, many of us are wrapped up in this and experiencing a lot of daily emotional turmoil over it. We look in the mirror and it reminds us that we aren't as thin as we used to be. We take our clothes off and feel utterly unattractive. We see recent pictures of ourselves and cringe, or pictures from a long time ago and wonder what the hell went wrong. We face complete emotional breakdown every time we go shopping for clothes.

You must break out of this cycle. Every human being, roughly from age 30 onward, sees a decline in their physical appearance. We don't get increasingly attractive as we get older, and I use the phrase "depreciating asset" to describe physical beauty. It's actually somewhat of a curse to develop your self-esteem from having good looks, as this is bound to slowly and steadily slip away, driving you mad and making you feel less self-worth if that is what you have based your self worth on.

In relationships and even casual encounters, the primary determinant of your attractiveness is your level of self-confidence – I prefer the term self-worth. Your self-worth is primarily determined by your own feelings of accomplishment, your skill levels in certain trades, your financial or vocational power, your intelligence, your sense of humor, your religious affiliations, how generous you are, and just about any other thing that you can manage to feel proud of. While physical attributes are certainly a big player in that, they are far from the only player. If they were the only player, rich old men wouldn't be able to attract young, beautiful women. But they can. And the women actually DO find the older men to be attractive because they are attracted to a lot more than just physical characteristics. A man with great wealth, international recognition for his skills and intelligence, and more will have swagger and confidence that will make him beat out a broke guy with perfect abs who can barely complete a sentence nine times out of ten. Good looks can get you to the door, but they can't take you all the way through to the other side.

With women, good looks, in many circumstances, can get you through to the other side. But if you derive all of your self-confidence from how you look, you're in for a world of hurt. You are bound to only be attractive to men who only care about looks, and you're not going to look the way you do in your youth forever. Get ready for a long, painful descent into old age with lots of plastic surgery and insecurity culminating with getting traded in for a newer model. Hey, you baited someone with your looks. Your looks change, you lose your appeal.

Anyway, we could break this down and down and down, deconstructing every atom of why it's short-sighted and even perhaps foolish to put so much time, effort, and emphasis on your physical appearance. In short, if you attract someone with your physical beauty but haven't cultivated any other skills, abilities, value, or qualities – brace yourself for attracting shallow people who will become less and less interested in you over time.

This is obviously all a bunch of propaganda to get you to focus your efforts elsewhere. And redirecting your drive and ambition and perfectionist tendencies towards other pursuits. Find something else to put your time and effort into. You are unlikely to just ditch the health fanaticism without becoming fanatical about something else as a substitute.

Can you imagine how good you could become at something creative like art or music by devoting as much time and thought to it as you do weight, nutrition, and health?

What about redirecting all this time and effort towards a new business – bringing a unique service or product to the world? Can you even imagine how much freaking dinero you would be rolling in a decade from now if you put the amount of time and effort into it as you have the last decade over your health, diet, and body composition? My business was up 2061% in December of 2012 compared to December of 2009. And I'm a terrible business man with no real drive to become wealthy. I mostly just sell books for less than $10. A good friend of mine who is 32 years old is going to clear $4 Million this year selling a mole removal cream that he formulated in his basement after reading an article by Dr. Weil. And that's only working about 15 hours a week!

Or what if you just studied something that you really like as much as you do health? Knowledge is valuable, no matter what that knowledge is, if you develop enough of it. The person that inspired me to begin my formal study of health really caught my attention when he said…

"Study something for two hours a day, and you can become one of the world's leading experts in that subject in 7 years. Study something for 4 hours a day and you can become one of the world's leading experts in that subject in 4 years. Study something 8

*hours a day and you can become one of the world's leading
authorities on that subject in just 2 years."*
~John Demartini

Or at least that's what I thought he said. Maybe
my numbers are screwed up, but that's the gist of it.

Of course, you have to really like and be
interested in what you are doing to do it enough to
actually obtain sought-after knowledge and talent. The
most important thing is that you spend your time doing
exactly what you want to be doing instead of obsessing
over your health and diet. I don't think you'll regret
becoming anything from a world class violinist or
millionaire to a movie trivia buff or a better parent by
redirecting your attention to something besides your
looks and macronutrient breakdown. And I can
virtually guarantee that you will get better quality and
quantity ▬▬ if you become distinguishably wealthy,
knowledgeable, or skilled somehow – if that's what
you're doing all those crunches and juice fasts for (I
doubt you are, but this still needed to be pointed out).

All this boiled down to just bare bones:

To fully recover from over-intellectualizing your
diet and health practices…

To fully recover from being chronically worried
about your health or your weight…

You must find something to replace this fixation.
Health fanaticism and body obsession operates like an
addiction. There is no substitute for, well, a substitute.
If you can find something, ideally something that you
are naturally interested in or compelled to do (like learn
an instrument or leave your husband or travel the world
or all of the above), and do the absolute hell out of it

with all your heart, soul, and passion – you have a much higher chance at true, lasting success with this. If you are bored and living an uninteresting and uninspired life, well, it's going to be tough not to just keep on thinking the same repetitive and neurotic thoughts about what you are eating or what your body fat percentage is today.

A garden overflows with weeds if you don't plant something in it. Actually putting a bunch of flowers and juicy tomatoes in there prevents the pests from popping up and taking over your life. Fill your life with what you want it full of, or it will fill up with annoying crap that gets in your way.

And for perhaps the most important part, really make sure, just like with your diet and health practices, that what you start doing is exactly what YOU want to do. Not what you think you SHOULD do based on moral obligations or self-loathing, not what someone else wants you to do or thinks you should do, not even something you wish you could be, but something that is genuinely and authentically you and yours.

Follow the path of least resistance yet again, and do exactly what is most interesting and inspiring at any given time, and follow through on your impulses. Spend time doing something you always loved but have gotten away from due to other obligations getting in the way. Do something that others had to peel you away from. Do something that others might think of as work but that you seem to be unable to get enough of. It's different for absolutely everyone. But you should be MORE you, not LESS you by not taking on someone else's dreams or trying to obtain something that someone else has out of envy or idolatry. If it's easy and effortless and takes no motivation whatsoever for you to do it – while it takes motivation to do things that aren't it, then you've found the right thing to immerse yourself in. And no it's not static. It changes and transforms and meanders. Follow it.

Okay okay, enough already with this motivational speech crap. If I lay it on any thicker I'll get nauseous proofreading it. And then I won't be able to eat enough to keep my metabolism up, hardy har har.

Best of luck everyone with turning to a new chapter in your life. You may have spent the last 10 to 20 years, maybe even longer, in an abusive and overly-analytical relationship with yourself, food, and more. Break out of that pattern, and revisit this book and my website as often as you need to for support and reassurance (for a while, then you shouldn't read ANY health-related information!). You don't want the next chapter of your life spent just like the last. And you don't want even the small amount of time and money invested in this book spent in vain, with everything I've shared fading away into the distant corners of your mind only to be eclipsed by the next late night infomercial.

(Was going to write a few more sentences, but ending it with the word "infomercial" was just too awesome – and these words don't count, they're in parentheses… Yes I know I use too many parentheses, you told me that already gosh!).

FAQ

Here are some of the refeeding questions I get most frequently, and my best answer for them...

You used to recommend eating only whole foods. Now you seem to think people should just eat whatever, including GMO's, high-fructose corn syrup, and other unhealthy things. Why is that? And is there anything wrong with eating "clean" during this process?

I think eating healthy, nutritious, chemical-free, and wholesome foods is great. If you can eat unrefined, wholesome foods and see your metabolic rate increase, you are doing well in all of the basic metabolism competencies (sex, digestion, sleep, warm hands and feet, etc.), and this feels like a realistic and sustainable way for you to eat – then by all means eat as puritanically as you desire.

But this is really more a matter of prioritization. For most people I think it is more freeing to just eat "normal," and that unshackling trumps minor concerns about the quality of the food being consumed.

For those in dire metabolic condition, calories are the most important single factor, and eating a rather uninspiring diet of unrefined, low-calorie density foods, is just not as effective — sometimes not effective at all or even counterproductive.

Other factors most do not consider is the fact that digestion is often very weak when metabolism is low, and the more refined and processed and pulverized and pureed a food is — the better it is digested and metabolized into real, usable, healing energy. Coarse, fibrous, and unrefined food may even worsen bacterial overgrowth in the small intestine and further exacerbate symptoms and slow metabolism. The high water content of the quintessential health foods is another factor than can inhibit metabolism increase.

Ultimately, most people don't need to think about the quality of their food or nutritional content to succeed, so I left almost all discussion about that completely out of the conversation. Heal first. Get all of your food demons exorcised from your conscience. Then maybe clean up your diet a little bit for a healthy and sustainable future.

I gained a lot of weight during refeeding, but it finally stopped after about six months. The weight is not coming off though, what should I do?

Have you tried going gluten-free? Nutri-System? Just kidding. Be patient. I know that excess body fat is uncomfortable and limits your ability to thrive physically. I don't carry suitcases around with me everywhere I go either, because nobody likes to carry around more weight than they have to. But if you gain a bunch of weight refeeding and then plunge yourself into another diet, then all you've done is basically complete the binge portion of the yo-yo dieting cycle.

Except now that you are aware of how to read your metabolic feedback, you won't be able to consciously violate your metabolism as hard as you used to, and you are even more likely to give up and just eat what you want than you were during your dieting days.

When men during World War II were starved for scientific study, they dieted for just a measly 24 weeks, then gained weight for 33 weeks, then maintained for a little while, and then weight slowly started coming off of them again – naturally and spontaneously. After 58 weeks, they were still dropping some body fat but still had not reached their level of leanness before the experiment began. These are healthy, high-metabolic men in their 20's and 30's we're talking about here, and their reaction to just one 24-week diet with roughly 1600 calories per day.

So I would expect to stick with it AT LEAST that long, if not longer, and continue to focus on keeping metabolic rate at maximum levels.

If you are going to do anything differently, I would say to put greater focus on your fitness and strength levels, making sure to avoid doing too much to jeopardize the high resting metabolism you've fought (well, if you call eating Tiramisu and sleeping a fight) so hard to achieve. The most important thing though, is patience and consistency.

If you can't resist the temptation to do traditional dieting (you are too vain and weak-minded), at least track your body temperature and do brief refeeds for one to two days every time you see a dip in morning body temperature or feel greater coldness creeping over your body – similar to the weight loss method described in obesity researcher Amanda Sainsbury-Salis's book *The*

Don't Go Hungry Diet. If you notice that it takes several weeks to lose 5 pounds, but only a few days to gain 10 back, well, you're screwed. Don't say I didn't warn you. *I have been refeeding and at first I was super hungry but now I don't have much of an appetite anymore. Should I just try to force it down?*

If you obey your appetite, or lack thereof, and the metabolism just comes crashing down and stays lowered for several weeks without rebound... then yes, force it down. But ultimately it would be great for everyone who follows this program to really get increasingly in tune with natural appetite cues, and eat EXACTLY how much food they desire EXACTLY when they desire it. Just as eating very little makes us compensate and eat a lot for a while, sometimes eating a lot will make you compensate and eat very little for a while. Not eating much isn't necessarily a diet if you're not hungry. I would just be careful with this reliance on internal cues if you have a serious history of eating disorders. Sometimes it's best to just eat in a programmed, machine-like way for a while and not have to even think about when, what, or how much you are eating – thinking about such things being a great source of anxiety for those with an eating-disordered past.

At first I felt great, but now I have been having headaches, trouble sleeping, feeling really tired, and just don't feel as well. Is there anything I should be doing differently?

You can overdo anything, including rest and refeeding, which is really meant to be a temporary strategy to push you back into a normal, balanced state more quickly. You might consider adding in more nutritious, higher-water content foods at this point. Nothing extreme, just adding in a few more. Drink more fluids and start sipping a little water throughout the day. Get more exercise and be more physically and mentally engaged. Don't force down cheesecake after two cheeseburgers if you already feel full and don't want to spend the next several hours in a mild food coma. Continue eating well throughout the day but maybe eat a little lighter in the evening when metabolism is already peaking. Little things like this may help to put you back into a balanced state, but this should be a good lesson for everyone as the body is not a static system. What works today may not work tomorrow. You have to be flexible and not tied to any one way of thinking/eating. Including this one. The perfect medicine to restore your health may be contraindicated for maintaining your health and vice versa.

Rest and Refeeding has gone great! But I started exercising recently after taking a few months off and I felt cold, my body temperature dropped, and I can't sleep again. Does this mean I'm not ready for exercise yet? And if not, how will I know when I am ready?

Just like radically changing your diet overnight, the body must be acclimated to what you are doing. If you haven't exercised in months and then get in even a light workout it can trigger a massive stressful revolt. Don't be too discouraged by this, but start out even more minimally and work on slow progress. I think almost everyone should exercise, and be doing something to build and maintain strength and fitness.

But you have to go slow and work within your limitations, not follow some regimen laid out by someone else with different limitations. This is of course why exercise programs and techniques devised by the fitness models, bodybuilders, and pro athletes that dominate the fitness industry don't do much for regular folk, and make naturally less rugged and out-of-shape folks sick, injured, and overtrained.

I hear that nuts and seeds and avocado have a lot of polyunsaturated fats in them. Ray Peat and others say to strictly avoid them. Is it okay to have some or not?

I personally haven't experienced any miracles from strictly avoiding polyunsaturated fats for an extended period of time (over a year), and know plenty of people that actually do better eating a lot of these types of fats. I wouldn't worry about it, but be very moderate about any of your dietary pursuits. As long as you aren't eating French fries and fried chicken for every meal and Doritos and peanut butter crackers for every snack you're on the right track. Like I said earlier, use real butter and coconut oil in your home cooking and you've already made a big improvement to your overall diet with virtually no sacrifice or thought whatsoever. That's the kind of change most people in seek of diet recovery need – not another firm set of "good" and "bad" foods.

Appendix I – Recommended Reading

While the ultimate is to start reading about a totally different subject entirely, immersing yourself into this new subject with gusto and passion, there are several books and websites that reiterate some of the things said in this book.

In a world where dieting, weight loss, health, and nutrition is coming in from all sides like a violent hailstorm, sometimes it helps to immerse yourself in the other side of the story. That other side of the story is not just in one book or website, but in over a hundred. I won't list them all here, but here are a few of the top sources for information that reinforces much of what has been written in *Diet Recovery 2*. Before you rush to buy all of them, 180DegreeHealth is currently working on a project to combine as many of these resources as possible in one affordable bundle, which we hope will be available by New Years of 2014…

Metabolism

Hypothyroidism: The Unsuspecting Illness by Broda Barnes
Hypothyroidism Type II: The Epidemic by Mark Starr
www.raypeat.com
www.dannyroddyweblog.com
www.eastwesthealing.com
www.andrewkimblog.com

Diet and Weight Loss Criticism

Health at Every Size by Linda Bacon
The Obesity Myth by Paul Campos
Big Fat Lies by Glenn Gaesser
Losing It by Laura Fraser
Rethinking Thin by Gina Kolata
Fat?So! by Marilyn Wann
Starffed by Gwyneth Olwyn of www.youreatopia.com
(2013 release)
Intuitive Eating by Evelyn Tribole
Eat What You Love, Love What You Eat by Michelle May
Stop Dieting Now by Golda Poretsky
www.junkfoodscience.blogspot.com
http://www.margaretcho.com/2003/11/06/the-fuck-it-diet/
www.thefuckitdiet.com
www.billycraig.co.uk
Health at Every Size Community Resources (an incredible list of books and supportive materials): http://www.haescommunity.org/resources.php?rType=b

Body Image Support

Body Traps by Judith Rodin
The Body Image Workbook by Thomas Cash
You'd Be So Pretty If… by Dara Chadwick
Perfect Girls, Starving Daughters by Courtney Martin
When Women Stop Hating Their Bodies by Jane Hirschmann and Carol Munter
www.haescommunity.org

Appendix II – Checking Body Temperature

As a former Broda Barnes worshiper, I used to recommend taking armpit (axillary) temperature first thing in the morning just like he had his patients do, with a target of 97.8 to 98.2 just like him as well. But I'm all grown up now and have ideas and experience of my own. Take the temperature wherever you want, just be consistent. Good morning-temperature targets are 99 butthole, 98.6 oral, 98.0 armpit. I don't know anything about ears and foreheads and vaginas and stuff. I'm old-school I guess. Later in the day temperatures should rise above that.

Armpits are weird though, so I'm kinda steering people away from that now. Sometimes the left and right armpits are a full degree different. That doesn't scream accuracy to me. So go oral, rectal, or vaginal. Man that's fun to write. Here are the best times to gather useful temperature data…

•Take one temperature first thing upon waking (good way to track how your resting metabolism is changing in response to your interventions).

•Take another temperature about a half hour after each meal (helps you determine what time of day you tend to need more calorie-dense food, and also how to structure food and fluids to give them the net-warming effect – as your temperature should always rise in response to food… if it doesn't you're either strung out on adrenaline and crashing – which will go away so stick with it, or your meal has too many fluids in proportion to calories and salt).

•Take another right before you go to bed (if it crashes right before bed, probably a good idea to regularly eat a tasty snack about a half hour before you go to sleep, like a dish of ice cream and something salty like a few handfuls of popcorn).

Do this for a few days, and then just start taking a morning temperature for a while to make sure it is trending upward. It doesn't move in a straight line. It goes up and down and up and down – but generally you should see it moving in the right direction in a general sense.

Women should know that when you start your menstrual cycle your temperatures will drop by about .5 degrees F. Don't be alarmed by this or discouraged. This is normal. After ovulation, your temperature should jump up and be slightly higher than the ideal temp targets listed above.

To make sure your temperature readings aren't artificially low, I recommend warming up your thermometer in your hand or something warm first. You don't want to stick a cold thermometer somewhere or the thermometer itself will actually lower the temperature of the area you are testing.

Once you have warmed up the thermometer to close to body temperature, put it in the testing orifice, then let it sit for at least a half a minute or longer. Then turn the digital thermometer on (a cheap Vicks digital thermometer is as good as any) and get a reading.

If you catch yourself taking more than just a few temperature readings during the day, or taking your body temperature every single day beyond the first few weeks as you start experimenting with this, you might want to throw away your thermometer. It's a useful tool. It's not a license to become obsessive.

After a month or so you should start to know your body metabolically. You should know what having a perfect temperature feels like and when to eat a little more, when to rest a little more, etc. You shouldn't really need a thermometer anymore other than to just check in every once in a while to see if you've fallen off the deep end.

That is all. Have fun.

Oh wait, one more tip. If you use the thermometer in your butt, don't take an oral reading with it right after, heh heh. Or leave it lying around where your kids might pick it up and check their oral temperatures out of curiosity.

References (a few anyway)

As you know, most of the assertions made in this book (and all my books) are the result of a combination of research, experience, communication with others, and good, old-fashioned reality. Few things written in the book can be tied directly to a specific study or resource. But here are a few links, websites, and books that played a more central role in the conclusions I found to be appropriate for inclusion in this book…

Atkins, Robert. *Dr. Robert Atkins New Diet Revolution.* Avon Books, Inc.: New York, NY, 1992.

Bacon, Linda. *Health at Every Size.* Benbella Books: Dallas, TX, 2008.

Barnes, Broda. *Hypothyroidism: The Unsuspecting Illness.* Harper and Row: New York, NY, 1976

Barnes, Broda. *Solved: The Riddle of Heart Attacks.* Robinson Press: Fort Collins, CO, 1976

Barnes, Broda. *Hope for Hypoglycemia.* Robinson Press: Fort Collins, CO, 1978

Bieler, Henry. *Food is Your Best Medicine.* Random House: New York, NY, 1965.

Brownstein, David. *Overcoming Thyroid Disorders.* Medical Alternative Press: West Bloomfield, MI, 2008.

Campos, Paul. *The Obesity Myth*. Gotham Books: New York, NY, 2004.

Chilton, Floyd H. *Inflammation Nation*. Fireside: New York, NY, 2007.

Farris, Russell and Per Marin. *The Potbelly Syndrome*. Basic Health Publications: Laguna Beach, CA, 2006.

Fife, Bruce. *Eat Fat Look Thin*. Healthwise: Colorado Springs, CO, 2002.

Fife, Bruce. *The Coconut Oil Miracle*. Avery: New York, NY, 1999.

Keys, Ancel et al. *The Biology of Human Starvation*. The University of Minnesota Press:
Minneapolis, MN, 1950.

Kharrazian, Datis. *Why Do I Still Have Thyroid Symptoms?* Morgan James Publishing: Garden City, NY, 2010.

Kolata, Gina. *Rethinking Thin*. Farrar, Straus and Giroux: New York, NY, 2007.

Langer, Stpehen E. and James F. Scheer. *Solved: The Riddle of Illness*. McGraw Hill: New York, NY, 2006.

Martin, Courtney E. *Perfect Girls, Starving Daughters*. Free Press: New York, NY, 2007.

Murray, Michael. *The Encyclopedia of Healing Foods*. Atria Books: New York, NY, 2005.

Page, Melvin, and H. Leon Abrams. *Health vs. Disease*, The Page Foundation, Inc., St. Petersburg, FL 1960.

Peat, Ray. *Progesterone in Orthomolecular Medicine*. Raymond Peat: Eugene, OR, 1993.

Peat, Ray. *Generative Energy*. Raymond Peat: Eugene, OR, 1994.

Peat, Ray. *Nutrition for Women*. Raymond Peat: Eugene, OR, 1993.

Peat, Ray. *Mind and Tissue*. Raymond Peat: Eugene, OR, 1993.

Peat, Ray. *From PMS to Menopause*. Raymond Peat: Eugene, OR, 1993.

Pool, Robert. *Fat: Fighting the Obesity Epidemic*. Oxford University Press: New York, NY, 2001.

Price, Weston A. *Nutrition and Physical Degeneration*. Republished by the Price-Pottenger Nutrition Foundation: La Mesa, CA, originally published in 1939.

Reaven, Gerald. *Syndrome X*. Fireside: New York, NY, 2000.

Rooney, Ric. *Secrets of a Professional Dieter* (eBook). www.PhysiqueTransformation.com

Ross, Julia. *The Diet Cure*. Penguin Books: New York, NY, 1999.

Schwartz, Bob. *Diets Don't Work!* Breakthrough Publishing: Houston, TX, 1982.

Schwarzbein, Diana. *The Schwarzbein Principle*. Health Communications, Inc.: Deerfield Beach, FL, 1999.

Schwarzbein, Diana. *The Schwarzbein Principle II*. Health Communications, Inc.: Deerfield Beach, FL, 2002.

Schwarzbein, Diana. *The Program*. Health Communications, Inc.: Deerfield Beach, FL, 2004.

Selye, Hans. *The Stress of Life*. McGraw-Hill: New York, NY, 1976.

Sears, Al. *P.A.C.E.* Wellness Research and Consulting, Inc.: Royal Palm Beach, FL, 2010.

Sears, Barry. *Enter the Zone*. Regan Books: New York, NY, 1995.

Sears, Barry. *The Age-Free Zone*. Regan Books: New York, NY, 1999.

Sears, Barry. *The Anti-Inflammation Zone*. Collins: New York, NY, 2005.

Sears, Barry. *Toxic Fat*. Thomas Nelson Inc, 2008.

Shell, Ellen Ruppel. *The Hungry Gene*. Atlantic Monthly Press: New York, NY, 2002.

Shomon, Mary J., *The Thyroid Diet*. Harper Resource: New York, NY, 2004.

Sisco, Pete. *Train Smart*. www.precisiontraining.com: 2012

Starr, Mark. *Hypothyroidism Type II*. Mark Starr Trust: Columbia, MO, 2005.

Talbott, Shawn. *The Cortisol Connection*. Hunter House: Alameda, CA, 2007.

Taubes, Gary. *Good Calories, Bad Calories*. Alfred A. Knopf: New York, NY, 2007.

Tribole, Evelyn and Elyse Resch. *Intuitive Eating*. St. Martin's Press: New York, NY, 1995.

Wann, Marilyn. *Fat!So?* Ten Speed Press: Berkeley, CA, 1998.

Wiley, T.S. *Lights Out: Sleep, Sugar, and Survival*. Pocket Books: New York, NY,
2000.

General Websites...

www.raypeat.com
www.youreatopia.com
www.dannyroddy.com
www.andrewkimblog.com
www.thefuckitdiet.com
www.haescommunity.org
www.eastwesthealing.com
www.chiefrok.com/blog
www.billycraig.co.uk
www.junkfoodscience.blogspot.com
www.carbsanity.blogspot.com

Specific Articles

"Seizures and Hypothermia due to dietary water intoxication in infants"
http://www.ncbi.nlm.nih.gov/pubmed/3563573?dopt=Abstract

"Association between obesity and reduced body temperature in dogs"
http://www.nature.com/ijo/journal/v35/n8/full/ijo2010253a.html

"Specific Gravity to Brix Conversion Table"
http://www.winning-homebrew.com/specific-gravity-to-brix.html

"Hyponatremia"
http://en.wikipedia.org/wiki/Hyponatremia

"Restoring Blood Volume"
http://www.ncbi.nlm.nih.gov/pmc/articles/PMC1701158/pdf/brmedj02
298-0064a.pdf

"The mysterious origins of the '8 glasses of water a day' rule"
http://www.mindthesciencegap.org/2012/10/22/you-need-to-drink-8-
glasses-of-water-a-day-a-history-lesson/

"Thyroid Disease and the Heart"
http://circ.ahajournals.org/content/116/15/1725.full

"Low urinary sodium is associated with greater risk of myocardial
infarction among treated hypertensive men"
http://www.ncbi.nlm.nih.gov/pubmed?term=%22Hypertension%22%5B
Jour%5D+AND+1995%5Bpdat%5D+AND+urinary+sodium&TransSc
hema=title&cmd=detailssearch

"Fatal and Nonfatal Outcomes, Incidence of Hypertension, and Blood
Pressure Changes in Relation to Urinary Sodium Excretion"
http://jama.jamanetwork.com/article.aspx?articleid=899663

"Water: swelling, tension, pain, fatigue, aging"
http://raypeat.com/articles/articles/water.shtml

"Salt, Energy, Metabolic Rate, and Longevity"
http://raypeat.com/articles/articles/salt.shtml

"TSH, temperature, pulse rate, and other indicators in hypothyroidism"
http://raypeat.com/articles/articles/hypothyroidism.shtml

"Coconut Oil"
http://raypeat.com/articles/articles/coconut-oil.shtml

"Water Intoxication"
http://en.wikipedia.org/wiki/Water_intoxication
"It's Time to End the War on Salt"

http://www.scientificamerican.com/article.cfm?id=its-time-to-end-the-war-on-salt

"What is Your Temperature? Rethinking 98.6"
http://well.blogs.nytimes.com/2009/12/28/whats-your-temperature-rethinking-986/

"Anorexia Nervosa and Eating Disorders"
http://medtextfree.wordpress.com/2010/09/03/anorexia-nervosa-and-eating-disorders/

The Female Athlete Triad Series at www.suppversity.blogspot.com   .

"Body Size, Energy Metabolism, and Lifespan"
http://jeb.biologists.org/content/208/9/1717.full

"Beneficial metabolic effects of regular meal frequency on dietary thermogenesis, insulin sensitivity, and fasting lipid profiles in healthy obese women"
http://ajcn.nutrition.org/content/81/1/16.abstract

"Rapid carbohydrate loading after a short bout of near maximal-intensity exercise"
http://www.ncbi.nlm.nih.gov/pubmed/12048325

"Small Mammal Metabolic Rates: Effect of Body Mass on Mass-Specific Metabolic Rate and Whole Animal Metabolic Rate"
http://www.franklincollege.edu/pwp/lmonroe/Metabolic%20Rate%20Lab.pdf

"A High Hypothalamus Diet"
http://www.economist.com/blogs/babbage/2012/03/obesity-and-brain?fsrc=scn/tw/te/bl/ahighhypothalamusdiet

"Top Off Breakfast with – Chocolate Cake?"
http://www.aftau.org/site/News2?page=NewsArticle&id=15967

"Nibbling vs. Gorging: Metabolic Advantages of Increased Meal Frequency"
http://www.nejm.org/doi/pdf/10.1056/NEJM198910053211403

"Impact of reduced meal frequency without caloric restriction on glucose regulation in healthy, normal-weight middle-aged men and women"
http://www.ncbi.nlm.nih.gov/pubmed/17998028

"Breakfast Reduces Chance of Obesity"
http://www.nutraingredients.com/Research/Breakfast-reduces-chances-of-obesity

"Athletes and Iron Deficiency"
http://sportsmedicine.about.com/cs/nutrition/a/012604.htm

"Low Energy Availability in Female Athletes"
http://emedicine.medscape.com/article/312312-overview

"Obesity: 10 Things You Thought You Knew"
http://www.youtube.com/watch?v=Qk4UKD00aOo&feature=channel

About the Author

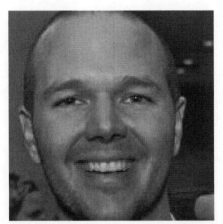

Matt Stone is an independent health researcher and author of more than 10 books on various health-related topics. He launched an independent investigation into health in 2005, and has since been exploring a wide range of health fields - from general physiology and nutrition to areas as diverse and specific as psychoneuroendocrinology. His investigation has yielded many great, practical insights and simple tips on how regular people can make substantial improvements in their health - for the purpose of both improving or eliminating specific health problems and preventing some of the most common ailments in the modern world. Most of his research has drawn him towards metabolic rate and how many basic functions (digestion, reproduction, aging, immunity, inflammation, sleep) perform better when metabolic rate is optimized.

Made in the USA
San Bernardino, CA
02 September 2013